Essential Oils

Essential oils are also known as volatile oils, ethereal oils, aetherolea, or simply as the 'oil of' the plant from which they are extracted, such as the oil of clove. An oil is 'essential' in the sense that it contains the characteristic fragrance of the plant that it is taken from. Essential oils do not form a distinctive category for any medicinal, pharmacological, or culinary purpose - and they are not essential for health, although they have been used medicinally in history. Although some are suspicious or dismissive towards the use of essential oils in healthcare or pharmacology, essential oils retain considerable popular use, partly in fringe medicine and partly in popular remedies. Therefore it is difficult to obtain reliable references concerning their pharmacological merits.

Medicinal applications proposed by those who sell or use medical oils range from skin treatments to remedies from cancer - and are generally based on historical efficacy. Having said this, some essential oils such as those of juniper and agathosma are valued for their diuretic effects. Other oils, such as clove oil or eugenol were popular for many hundreds of years in dentistry and as antiseptics and local anaesthetics. However as the use of essential oils has declined in evidence based medicine, older text-books are frequently our only sources for information! Modern works are less inclined to generalise; rather than referring to 'essential oils' as a class at all, they prefer to discuss specific compounds, such as methyl salicylate, rather than 'oil of wintergreen.'

Nevertheless, interest in essential oils has considerably revived in recent decades, with the popularity of aromatherapy, alternative health stores and massage. Generally, the oils are volatized or diluted with a carrier oil to be used in massage, or diffused in the air by a nebulizer, heated over a candle flame, or burned as incense. Their usage goes way back, and the earliest recorded mention of such methods used to produce essential oils was made by Ibn al-Baitar (1188-1248), an Andalusian physician, pharmacist and chemist. Different oils were claimed to have differing properties; some to have an uplifting and energizing effect on the mind such as grapefruit and jasmine, whilst others such as rose lavender have a reputation as de-stressing and relaxing - and also, usefully, as an insect repellent.

The oils themselves are usually extracted by 'distillation', often by using steam -but some other processes include 'expression' or 'solvent extraction'. Distillation involves raw plant material (be that flowers, leaves, wood, bark,

PRACTICAL HAND-BOOK

OF

TOILET PREPARATIONS

AND THEIR USES.

ALSO

RECIPES FOR THE HOUSEHOLD.

———

**FORMULAS THAT HAVE BEEN TESTED BY THE AUTHOR IN A
LONG PROFESSIONAL CAREER, WHICH WILL ENABLE THE
READER TO MAKE, AT A SMALL PRICE, A CLASS OF
PREPARATIONS THAT ARE IN UNIVERSAL DE-
MAND, AND ARE POSITIVELY HARMLESS.**

———

*The information contained in this Book is the result of original investi-
gations, and cannot be obtained in its entirety without a lifetime of research.*

———

BY

JOSEPH A. BEGY.

British Library Cataloguing-in-Publication Data
A catalogue record for this book is available from the
British Library

roots, seeds or peel) put into an alembic (distillation apparatus) over water. As the water is heated, the steam passes through the plant material, vaporizing the volatile compounds. The vapours flow through a coil, where they condense back to liquid, which is then collected in the receiving vessel. 'Expression' differs in that it usually merely uses a mechanical or cold press to extract the oil. Most citrus peel oils are made in this way, and due to the relatively large quantities of oil in citrus peel and low cost to grow and harvest the raw materials, citrus-fruit oils are cheaper than most other essential oils. 'Solvent extraction' is perhaps the most difficult of the three methods, and is generally used for flowers, which contain too little volatile oil to undergo expression. Instead, a solvent such as hexane or supercritical carbon dioxide is used to extract the oils.

These techniques have allowed essential oils to be used in all manner of products; from perfumes to cosmetics, soaps - and as flavourings for food and drinks as well as adding scent to incense and household cleaning products. The science, history and folkloric tradition of essential oils is incredibly fascinating - and a still much debated area. We hope the reader is inspired by this book to find out more.

"*Prove all things, and hold fast that which is good.*"

"*That which is new is attractive by the charm of its originality, and when possessing the undisputed advantage of practical usefulness, must and will call for admiration.*"

PREFACE.

In offering this work to the public my aim is to place before the people my formulas for making, with instructions for using, the different preparations for preserving, improving and beautifying the face, neck, arms, lips, teeth and hair; also for making a large variety of other preparations for toilet use and other purposes, so that my readers can secure for themselves the manifold advantages of my long experience.

There is no work that will stand higher in the estimation of the public or that will be more highly appreciated for the benefits received through it, when its merits shall become known.

A large number of my recipes are for making preparations that will perhaps to a large extent be used by the ladies, as they are adapted especially to their needs and wants. There are, however, many recipes, which are designed for gentlemen, who must also have toilet preparations for the face, after shaving, and for the hands, to prevent the skin becoming rough and chapped. Besides these, they will also find preparations for the teeth, hair, scalp, moustache, whiskers, etc. I have endeavored to make the matter in this work plain, so that everybody will be enabled to employ the different preparations made after my recipes in the most satisfactory manner, and with a thorough understanding of just what they are using. I have placed before the public the results of my extensive experimenting, and special study of the various articles, substances and materials used in making toilet preparations. During many years' experience as a druggist, I have given particular attention to this branch; and made a special study of the subject, in order to be able to supply my patrons with preparations that I knew to be perfectly reliable, safe, and sure to produce the effect desired in the shortest possible time. After long experimenting I succeeded in making a large number of preparations that have fulfilled all requirements. I therefore offer the results of my labors and experience with the utmost confidence that they will give entire satisfaction to everybody who uses them; for they have all been thoroughly tried, and will do just what I claim for them—preserve and beautify the complexion—soften and whiten the hands— give to the lips the fresh ruby condition denoting health —preserve and beautify the teeth—and impart beauty, strength and vigor to the hair. They are pronounced by competent judges to be wonderful combinations. Nobody can use them without being well pleased with the result.

In making a special study of toilet preparations, I

found that a great many so-called Beautifiers, Creams, Balms, Cosmetics, Lotions, Invigorators, Restoratives, Tonics, and powders and paste preparations, with all manner of names, that flood the market, contain deleterious materials, and should never be used, as they often prove very detrimental to health. But those who use my recipes and follow the directions, will have the advantage of knowing that they contain positively no deleterious material, and are perfectly harmless. This can only be known by my formulas, which show the nature of the materials used.

This is a subject every one who uses toilet preparations, in some form, (and who does not?) for the face, hands, lips, teeth, arms, neck and hair, should be interested in. Very often serious consequences follow the use of these highly lauded preparations, and if their actual nature were known they would be discarded. But how little attention has the purity of these preparations received? It has been almost overlooked in the great desire to get something that seemed to serve the purpose for the time being, regardless of consequences.

My special study of this subject enables me to place before the public, in this work, formulas for making the various toilet preparations that are absolutely free from all injurious substances—and are equal or superior to the best now before the public. I have also placed in this work formulas for making a great many useful, practical and valuable preparations for family use other than the toilet.

There need be no hesitation whatever in using any of the preparations made after these recipes, as they are positively reliable, and will generally do just what is claimed for them, producing results that never fail to please.

Trusting that this work will, by its merits, prove worthy of public confidence, I respectfully submit it to the test of experience.

JOSEPH A. BEGY.

Rochester, N.Y., August 1, 1889.

RECIPES AND PREPARATIONS FOR TOILET AND HOUSEHOLD USE.

A FEW THINGS I HAVE OBSERVED.

I HAVE observed that anything that has the appearance of mystery will arouse the curiosity of a multitude of people.

This is the very secret of success with a great many of the so-called wonderful preparations that to-day are being lauded to the skies by the extensive use of money and printer's ink.

If the mask were taken off of these preparations, and the true nature of their composition exposed, it would result in their certain death.

During my long experience as a druggist I have come in contact a great deal with an article called humbug.

I have been repeatedly and forcibly reminded of the fact that there are some people who love to be imposed upon, when it is done without their direct knowledge.

All that is necessary to prove this assertion is to take notice how some preparations are placed before the public, being surrounded with all the mysterious conditions that the parties were able to contrive. If such success follows preparations that depend largely on mystery, how much greater should be the success of a work like this that comes to the people with recipes, that every pharmacopolist can understand—formulas written in plain language and based on scientific principles ; thus I obtain results that are in keeping with established laws. If any reader should infer that ingredients apparently so simple and common are not efficacious, he will in their use be agreeably surprised.

The mixing together of different ingredients in the proper proportions and blending of materials produces wonderful combinations.

To all who are sceptical I wish to say, do not condemn the work until you have tried its merits.

My recipes are not merely a random compilation, but are the outgrowth of deep study of the subject backed up by thorough practical experimenting, until the most effective preparations were produced.   This has been demonstrated by having them thoroughly tried during my many years' service as a druggist.

Preparations made after a recipe that the people can know all about, will take the place of noxious concoctions disguised under fancy names.   For it must be a matter of considerable satisfaction to anybody to have full knowledge of the constituents of any preparation used on the person.

If this work only partially accomplishes the aims I have had in view, and consigns to oblivion the noxious compounds sold for personal use, I shall feel that my labor has not been lost.

J. A. B.

THE SKIN.

HOW TO PRESERVE AND IMPROVE ITS VELVETY TEX-
TURE AND THE DELICACY OF ITS HUES.

THIS is a subject that will no doubt interest the
ladies very much.

In order to be successful in such an undertaking, it
is very necessary to follow certain rules. The skin
must be protected as much as possible from vigorous
exposure, and from all extreme influences that might
have a tendency to affect it injuriously.

Do not put on any preparations except those you
know contain no injurious substances.

Do not expose the hands, arms, neck or face to extreme heat or cold, nor to sudden and extreme changes
of temperature, for the vicissitudes of weather and climate have a tendency to destroy the natural sensibility
of the skin; to thicken and harden it; to render it
coarse and rough, thereby causing the obstruction and
rupture of the capillary arteries, and imparting to it a
streaky, muddy, weather-beaten appearance.

Strong winds, whether hot or cold, also prove very
injurious, by carrying off most of the natural moisture
which is essential to its suppleness and proper action.

This very often, by repeated exposure, is carried to a
degree sufficient to destroy its vitality, and even to
produce an ugly, rough, red and chapped condition of
the skin, which at times becomes sore, painful and un-

sightly—a condition that often becomes a difficult problem to successfully handle and to cure.

To obviate the ill effects of exposure and to promote the beauty of the skin, the assistance of art is frequently had recourse to ; when such is the case, bear in mind, it should be done in the most judicious manner, and with utmost caution.

Generally, all that is necessary, under ordinary circumstances, for this purpose, are the following rules :

If the health has been impaired by the use of any deleterious toilet preparations or from other causes, this should first be restored.

Discontinue the use of the toilet preparations that contain the injurious material, and in their place employ the different preparations made after the recipes in this work.

No matter what the blemishes may be, or what character they assume, or that your skin may be affected with, this book contains the recipes for making preparations that will, by proper use, remove all blemishes from the skin, giving to it that fine, velvety texture, and healthy, fair, youthful appearance so much admired, and so highly coveted by all.

This very desirable condition of the skin can be produced very readily with the aid of this work.

The modus operandi is to follow the rules here laid down, and to use the different preparations for the skin and toilet made after my recipes, carefully following the instructions. The results will justify my confidence in what they will do, when used according to my suggestions.

In bathing the face, neck, arms and hands, always

use soft water when it can be had, as hard water renders the skin rough and coarse, gradually destroying its natural beauty. But hard water can be rendered fit to use by the addition of a little aqua ammonia or pulverized borax.

In the following pages you will find a recipe for making what I call " Bathing Powder." This is one of the very finest preparations for rendering hard water soft ; after this has been added to the hardest water, it will render it soft and fit for people to use, who have the most tender and delicate skin. It is an excellent wash for salt rheum, and many other skin diseases. The addition of this powder to water will in no way be incompatible with the soap you use.

It is very important to be particular about the quality of soap. Do not use any but the very purest.

Purity of quality should be the standard and watchword of everybody for everything used upon the skin, as impure or deleterious materials will prove injurious and cause no end of suffering from irritation and inflammation of the skin.

When you find, after using the preparation you have selected, that it don't agree with the skin, reduce it ; if too weak make it stronger, or use one that is heavier. It is well, however, to keep in mind the fact that very few preparations will act alike on any great number of people ; with some a preparation might agree in every respect, while with others this same preparation would prove very unsatisfactory.

Consequently, when one is used that does not prove satisfactory, use another until the right one is found.

This book contains a large number of different

preparations for the skin, among which, no doubt one will be found that will more than meet your expectations.

A great aid in receiving the most satisfactory results in the employment of the various preparations for beautifying the skin is to have the blood in a pure state; it is often in such bad condition as materially to hinder a cure. I would suggest the use of some good medicine when necessary to get the blood in a purer state. I have given recipes for making preparations, by the use of which this can generally be accomplished.

HOW AND WHERE TO PROCURE THE MATERIALS FOR MAKING THE DIFFERENT PREPARATIONS IN THIS BOOK.

READ THIS CAREFULLY.

WHEN you desire to procure the materials, or to have any of these preparations prepared, copy the recipe you desire to use, and go to any good drug-store and either get the ingredients and prepare it yourself, or else have your druggist put it up for you.

There will be no difficulty whatever in procuring any of the articles called for in the various formulas at any good drug-store.

It is very important, in buying any of the materials used, to secure only the very best, freshest and purest goods.

When the recipe calls for articles in powder form it must be in the very finest powder. All oils used should be fresh and of best quality, and in like manner everything used in making the preparations after my recipes must be pure and fresh in order to get satisfactory results in every respect.

You can get just the amount that any of the recipes calls for, or if you wish the amount can be reduced or increased; but keep the proportions the same as in the formula.

When the recipe you may select makes a larger quantity than you wish to try, reduce it to such a quantity as will suit; and when you find the quantity is not large enough increase it to the amount you wish.

It will be well, however, to keep in mind the fact that a small quantity will in most instances cost almost as much as a larger quantity. The prices of a good many of the articles used are very low; especially is this the case when they are bought in fair quantities.

When the above course is followed, first-class preparations will be the result, and their effect will not disappoint you, as perhaps many ready-made preparations have done, though put in nice looking bottles or boxes, all finely labelled with a very plausible tale of their wonderful properties, and of the great transformation that would take place after they have been used.

With this work to make your preparations from, there will be no question about what they are composed of, and the cost will be far below these patented and inferior wares.

When we consider the price charged for goods of this character, there can be no question about the value of this work. By its aid you can make your own toilet and various other preparations at decidedly less expense than the preparations which are generally sold for similar purposes.

The preparations made after my formulas will invariably give satisfaction when prepared strictly according to instructions. Do not fail to try them.

A FEW WORDS TO THE LADIES.

Ladies, allow me to submit for your inspection the following suggestions:

Follow the instructions laid down in this book, and use my preparations for completing the toilet and the various other purposes mentioned, and there will be no further occasion to find fault because the toilet preparations you use for the face, neck, arms, hands, lips, teeth and hair have disappointed you. My colognes, toilet waters and numerous other preparations used in completing the toilet never fail to give satisfaction.

There will be no more cause for alarm on account of the serious consequences which followed the use of some of the highly injurious toilet preparations which are advertised as perfectly harmless.

There is no question about the fact that a great many ladies are daily using preparations for their complexions and toilet that are more or less injurious; they will not realize what danger they are in until some day they find that they have completely ruined their skin. This will cause them no end of chagrin.

If they were acquainted with the nature of the materials, they would not sanction their use. Hitherto there has been no choice, they could only take such preparations as were offered (generally at exorbitant prices), and run the risk of good or bad results. With this book in your possession that will all be changed; you will not have to take anything offered or go

2

without; but will have the matter completely under your own control; and be able to select and use only such preparations as you know to be not only harmless but beneficial.

This is a very important matter, and should not be lost sight of. I have placed before you a large number of useful recipes, both for toilet and household use, to make your selections from.

If the old adage is true that economy is wealth, it will be realized through this book in an exceedingly surprising manner, for you will be in a position to dispense with the preparations that are sold at such exorbitant prices, and in their place you can have yours made from my recipes at considerable less expense and with the assurance of guaranteed excellence; therefore I trust you will see the wisdom of the above suggestions and act accordingly, securing for yourselves beauty, health, contentment, comfort and happiness.

READ THE FOLLOWING CAREFULLY.

SPECIAL DIRECTIONS AND INSTRUCTIONS FOR USING PREPARATIONS MADE AFTER RECIPES IN THIS BOOK.

IT will be very important to have all the preparations you desire to use prepared correctly and from the very best materials.

Ladies using the toilet preparations in liquid form for the face, neck and arms, should apply them with a fine, soft sponge. After putting on the required amount (this your judgment must decide), *give it time to dry*; then take a soft piece of chamois skin and rub it over very lightly; this will smooth it over nicely and evenly. This must be done in order to produce the best effect, and one you will appreciate.

The above course should be followed in the use of all liquid preparations for preserving, improving and beautifying the complexion and skin (unless otherwise directed in the recipe.)

Any of the liquid preparations (or those in powder form), made after my recipes for the face, can also be used on the neck and arms with the most charming results.

They should be applied lightly, then allowed to dry; then rubbed over with fine chamois skin to smooth down evenly.

Ladies using any of the preparations in powder form should apply them with a soft chamois skin, cotton-flannel, or puff. Your judgment must decide the quantity that will be required to bring out the most desirable features.

When finished in this way, detection of its presence is very difficult. This is really one of the secrets of using toilet preparations for the face, and those using them should take advantage of it.

The one best adapted to your skin should be used.

There is a large number to choose from (and all good for their purpose); so there will be no difficulty to select those that will be perfectly satisfactory and suitable to the different tastes.

Always remember that the preparations must be put on even—not more on one place than on another.

A lady appearing with her toilet carelessly attended to, or with powder applied in a careless manner (as though done by an amateur), looks coarse and vulgar. But my preparations cannot be readily detected, when manipulated and applied, so as to bring out the most desirable features, when their natural freshness has faded. Less fascinating features are thus placed out of sight.

With this book, and a little intelligent practice, any one can be sure of success in the use of toilet preparations, providing the latter are what they should be. If you follow the instructions in this book you may be sure of appearing to as good advantage as any of your friends, perhaps completely surpass them.

There is no need whatever of having the face all covered with unsightly and disagreeable blemishes, the skin yellow, streaky, spotted or florid ; to allow time to leave his marks too soon upon the once fair face; to have the hands red or rough, the lips pale, feverish, cracked and chapped, or the teeth all discolored and decayed

The teeth above all things should be properly taken care of.

It is a conceded fact that good health depends upon cleanliness ; and where is the necessity more apparent than in the mouth ? A good dentifrice will keep the teeth and mouth in a cleanly condition, thereby preserving and beautifying the teeth, and promoting health, happiness, and beauty.

My recipes for preparations are equal, and many are far superior to any of the high priced preparations usually sold. I have given a large variety to select from, and there will be no difficulty in getting just the kind that may be desired.

Do not neglect the hair. If it does not receive proper attention, it soon becomes dry, harsh and coarse ; and the scalp will become covered with scaly matter, called dandruff, lose its vitality and turn prematurely gray, or fall out, causing baldness.

How often this happens, when it might have been prevented by proper care. Do not wait until the life of the hair has been destroyed, but take care of it while there is still a chance to preserve it.

By the use of the creams, balms, lotions, restoratives, tonics, invigorators, cosmetics, powders, and the various other preparations made from my recipes, the skin, teeth and hair will certainly be preserved, improved and beautified. They are truly efficacious preparations and such will be the verdict of all who employ them.

Gentlemen desiring preparations to use after shaving, to prevent the face becoming rough and chapped, will find in this book a number of recipes adapted to their use. It also contains formulas for making Hair Tonics, Restorers, Invigorators, Shampoos, Brilliantin, Dyes, Curling Fluid, and Dressing through which the hair can be brought to a degree of perfection that is simply wonderful.

Ladies or gentlemen desiring any of the various Toilet Waters, Colognes, or Bay Rums, can find recipes in this book to make those that will be equal to any of the imported or domestic, in elegance, fragrance, and lasting qualities, so that the most exacting person will be well suited with them.

There are a great many preparations in the market

put up for similar purposes, which sell at exorbitant prices, that cannot compare with those made from my recipes in actual results.   A trial of them will convince the most sceptical.

I trust you will be confirmed in the truthfulness of the statements made above by buying this work and giving the preparations made after my recipes a trial.

I am confident that after they are once used, they will be the favorite ones, and that this work will be appreciated.

THE DESIRE TO BE BEAUTIFUL

is one of the most praiseworthy, as well as the most natural sentiments of a woman's heart.

There can be no real beauty without a pure complexion and clear skin.

Any lady can have this by using the preparations for the skin and complexion made after the formulas in this book.

PART I.

PREPARATIONS FOR BEAUTIFYING THE COMPLEXION AND SKIN.

"TOKALON,"

FOR IMPROVING AND BEAUTIFYING THE COMPLEXION.

This makes an elegant preparation. It imparts a brilliant transparency to the skin; it will remove pimples, freckles and discolorations, and make the skin delicately soft.

Best Precipitated Chalk, 4 ounces,
" Sub. Nitrate Bismuth, 1 ounce,
Pure Glycerine, 2 ounces,
Pulv. Carmine, 3 grains
Pulv. Borax, 1½ drachm,
Best Bay Rum, 4 ounces,
Extract Jockey Club, 4 drachms,
Water, 1 pint.

Mix all the ingredients together in a suitable bottle. Keep well corked.

Directions for using.

Shake thoroughly, then apply to the face, arms or neck. It improves the effect to thoroughly wash; then dry the parts before applying the Tokalon. It should be put on lightly with a small sponge; when nearly dry rub even with soft cloth or chamois skin.

ORANGE CREAM

FOR THE COMPLEXION.

This preparation produces a beautiful effect upon

the skin; it renders it soft and smooth; it will also allay smarting, caused by sunburn and other irritation of the surface.

Take

    Pulv. White Venetian Talcum, 3 ounces,
    Pulv. Drop Chalk, 1 ounce,
    Pure Glycerine, 1½ ounce,
    Bicarbonate Soda, 2 drachms,
    Extract musk, 2 drachms,
    Oil Sweet Orange, ½ drachm,
    Alcohol, ½ ounce,
    Pure water, 1 pint.

Prepare by adding the powders to the water, then add the glycerine and extract. Dissolve the oil in the alcohol and add it to the other ingredients.

This cream may be used upon the skin just as desired, and as often as desired. Apply it with soft sponge or cloth. Do not put it on too thick.

MAIDEN BLUSH

FOR THE COMPLEXION.

This is a beautiful, highly-tinted preparation.

It imparts such a natural appearance to the complexion, it is very much admired.

' The effect it produces is truly marvellous; it conceals all blemishes.

It can be blended with an all white preparation when applying it, so that it will bring out the very best effects.

When this is desired it may be done as follows:

Apply one of the all white preparations (in liquid form); allow it to become dry, and smooth over very lightly; then apply just enough of the Maiden Blush right over the white, to produce the desired effect.

Take

Best Precipitated Chalk, 2 ounces.
" Drop Chalk, 2 ounces.
Oxychlor, Bismuth, 2 drachms.
Pulv. Borax, 2 drachms.
Pure Carmine, 5 grains.
" Glycerine, 1½ ounce.
" Bay Rum, 2 ounces.
Extract Vanilla, 2 drachms.
" White Rose, 2 drachms.
" Jasmin, 1 drachm.
" Musk, 1 drachm.
Pure water to make one pint.

Put powders in a pint bottle; add the glycerine, Bay rum, extracts and water. Keep well corked.

Directions.

Apply to face, arms or neck as required; put on even; not too thick.

This makes a very desirable preparation for evening use, giving to the skin a natural, youthful appearance. It will at once change the color of the skin, no matter how badly it is freckled or sunburned; or if it has a sickly brown or yellowish appearance, this will at once change it to a beautiful becoming flesh tint. It is not easily detected on account of the natural hue it imparts to the skin.

"SNOW-DROP CREAM."

· FOR THE COMPLEXION, HANDS, NECK, AND ARMS.

This is an elegant creamy white preparation. I have always considered it one of the finest combinations I ever put together. If you want a creamy white toilet preparation that you can always rely upon, do not fail to try this one; it will not disappoint you. Take

Pulv. " Pure White " Talc, } each 3½ ounces.
 " " Precipitated Chalk, }
 " Oxychlor. Bismuth, 4 drachms.
 " Borax 2 "
Pure Glycerine, 1½ ounce.
Camphor water, 2 drachms.
Extract Lily of the Valley, 1 drachm.
 " Jockey Club, 2 drachms.
 " Frangipani, 2 drachms.
Pure water to make one pint. Mix powders all together, put into pint bottle, add the glycerne, extracts, camphor water, and lastly the plain water; shake together thoroughly.

Directions.

Always shake well before using; apply it as desired.

This preparation will be highly appreciated by those that desire to have a fair white complexion and skin.

This can also be blended with one of the liquid rouges to very good advantage.

Ladies should study blending; it will more then pay for the time occupied, in the result to be obtained.

"THE ARABIAN"

COMPLEXION BEAUTIFIER.

This preparation is of a peculiar color; it is therefor very much admired by people of the brunette type of beauty.

Take

Finely Pulverized Paris White, 2 ounces.
" White Talcum, 2 ounces.
Cherry Laurel water, 1½ "
Jamaica Rum, 2½ "
Pure. Glycerine, 1½ "
French Brandy, 1 oz.
Extract Jockey Club, 2 drachms.
" Ylang Ylang, 2 drachms.

Water to make one pint. Mix powders together; put into a pint bottle; then add other ingredients, and shake together well; then fill with water.

The ladies are the best judges as to how much and how often they should use their toilet preparations; it is a matter depending largely upon circumstances.

Generally they may be applied to the face, neck, arms, and hands as required.

CAPITAL TOILET CREAM

FOR THE COMPLEXION.

This makes a very elegant preparation; it is one that I have put up for a long time; it will at one change the color of the skin and impart to it a very refreshing soothing, healthy condition, and a delicate velvety appearance, very much admired.

Take

Pulv. Drop Chalk, 2 ounces.
" White French Chalk, 2 ounces.
" Sub Nitrate Bismuth, ½ ounce.
" Borax, 1 drachm.
Peppermint Water, 1 ounce.
Pure Glycerine, 1½ ounce.
Extract Ocean Spray, 3 ounces.
" Violets, 3 drachms.
Water enough to make one pint.

Prepare by mixing all the powders; then put them into a pint bottle; pour on the peppermint water and glycerine (which should be previously mixed); then add the extracts and lastly the water, and then shake well together.

Directions for using.

Shake well and apply as required; be particular about getting this on good, and the effects will surely be gratifying and wonderful. It cannot fail to be a favorite.

Any of the pure white (that is, the all-white) preparations in liquid form may be tinted, if desired, by adding a small quantity of the liquid rouge or of pure carmine to them.

Add just enough to produce the desired tint to suit your complexion and skin.

"PARISIAN EUREKA,"

FOR THE TOILET.

This recipe will make a preparation that is very soothing and healing to the skin; when the skin is rough or irritated, it works charmingly in allaying irritation and in curing roughness of the skin. Take

Pulv. Alum, 2 drachms.
Precipitated Chalk, 2½ ounces.
Sub Nitrate Bismuth, 2 ounces
Rose Water, 3 ounces.
Peppermint Water, 3 ounces.
New England Rum, 1 ounce.
Tinct. Benzoin, *plain*, ½ drachm.
Extract Heliotrope, 3 drachms.
Pure Water, 12 ounces.

Mix the powders, and the rose and peppermint waters, then the rum, extract heliotrope and Benzoin, and lastly the water ; shake together thoroughly. Put on evenly and not too thick.

PRACTICAL TOILET CREAM,

FOR THE COMPLEXION AND SKIN.

This preparation is thoroughly practical and an excellent one for everyday use. To be used as often as desired in all kinds of weather. Take

Best Paris White, 1½ ounce.
Pulv. White French Chalk, ½ ounce.
Precipitated Chalk, 2 ounces,
Pure Glycerine, 1 ounce.
Pulv. Borax, 2 drachms.
Extract Jockey Club, 2 drachms.
Bay Rum, 2 ounces.
Pure Water, 1 pint.

Mix powders ; put in suitable bottle and add all the other ingredients, the water last. This preparation may be tinted, if desired, by adding a little carmine.

Directions.

Shake well and apply as desired. Put on evenly, not too heavy. Applying it with a soft sponge ; allow

RED ROSE BALM.

This preparation will give to the complexion a very rosy hue. It will at once change the color of the skin from a yellow, sickly appearance to one of health and beauty. It especially delights the hearts of those who have a sallow, disagreeable looking skin.

Take

Pure Pulv. Drop Chalk, 4 ounces.
White Venetian Talc, ½ ounce.
Pure Carmine, 5 grains.
" Glycerine, 1 ounce.
Extract White Rose.
" Jockey Club, each, 2 drachms.
Aqua Ammonia, 2 drachms.
Pure Water, 14 ounces.

Prepare as follows:

Dissolve the carmine in the ammonia; mix the powders together, put into pint bottle; add the glycerine, extracts, and the solution of carmine, then the water, and shake all together thoroughly. Keep well corked.

Directions.

Shake well and apply with a soft sponge or cloth; allow it to dry, then rub it even with a soft piece of chamois skin.

Put on just enough to produce the desired effect.

"THE UNEXCELLED CREAM."

FOR THE SKIN,

I desire to call special attention to this preparation; it will be noticed that it differs very much in character as well as in effect from most of the preparations for the complexion. It is very much admired for its applicability to the skin. It is generally used with entire satisfaction. Those that have used it are enthusiastic in their praise of its qualities, it has such wonderful softening properties, through which it renders the skin smooth and transparent. It gives to it the appearance of youth on account of the delicate tint it bestows. I assure all who desire an extra fine preparation for the complexion, that this will meet their expectation and approval.

Its effect is immediate and more lasting than that of most other preparations.

This recipe makes an all-white preparation. Further on will be found instructions for tinting it to any shade desired.

Take

    Pure fresh Oil Sweet Almonds, 6 drachms,
      "   "   Cacao Butter, 4 drachms,
    Pulv. White French Chalk, 8 drachms,
    Sub Nitrate Bismuth, 2 drachms,
    Pure Precipitate Chalk, 1½ ounce,
    Pulv. Borax, 20 grains,
    Pure Glycerine, 2 drachms,
    Tinct. Benzoin, plain, 2 drachms,
    Oil Rose Geranium, 10 drops,
    " Bitter Almonds, 2   "
    Ottar Roses, 2 drops.
    Oil Bergamot, 8 drops.

HOW TO PREPARE THIS CREAM.

Directions for making the above should be followed very carefully, thereby assuring an elegant preparation that will suit the most exacting taste.

First take a suitable dish in which it can be prepared. In this place the Cacao butter; then heat it until it has melted; then add the oil of sweet almonds. When it has been incorporated, the powders (they must be previously mixed) should be added gradually to the oil and Cacao butter, stirring the mixture continually until all the powder has been added, then add the tincture Benzoin and the glycerine.

If the cream becomes too stiff before all the ingredients have been put in, apply a little heat; this will at once soften it; then proceed to add the remainder; after this has been done, add the oils geranium, bitter almonds, rose and bergamot. (These oils should be the last thing added in preparing the cream.) Then stir all together very thoroughly for a short time, it can be put into a suitable jar or box, in which it should be kept for use. The cream should always be well covered; this will preserve its delicious fragrance,

When the above recipe is properly prepared it makes a beautiful creamy paste which will remain on the skin better and longer then the majority of other preparations.

Directions for using the cream.

Apply to the skin with soft chamois skin and rub it on well, or take some of the paste on the flat part of middle finger, and rub it in very thoroughly. It can also be applied by taking soft sponge that has been previously moistened in warm water (do not have it too wet); rub the sponge over the paste lightly, then apply it to the skin and smooth over nicely.

If this cream is kept in a very warm place it is apt to become quite soft, or if it is kept in a very cold place it becomes very hard. By keeping it in a moderate temperature, the consistency will be just right to use easily.

TINTED CREAM FOR THE SKIN.

To give to "the unexcelled cream" a beautiful tint, imparts to the skin a color that will in every respect resemble so closely the natural color of vigorous youth, as to defy detection from the most scrutinizing observer.

A great many will take advantage of the effects of this preparation in order to retain their youthful appearance.

The recipe, whenever desired, may be modified to produce different degrees of tint, by adding a little more or less of the *solution of carmine.* I have most generally found that the following added to the cream will give satisfaction:

Take

Pure Carmine, 1 grain.
Aqua Ammonia, 1 drachm.

Dissolve the carmine in the ammonia; then add it to the cream just before the last oils are added. When the all-white cream is prepared, it may be heated just enough to warm it slightly, and then the carmine solution should be added; it must always be very thoroughly stirred, in order to have the color even throughout. When making the cream, half of it may be colored or tinted, and the other half left white; this can be done very easily. Make the cream as directed; when the white is all finished divide it into two parts, one of which may be tinted as above.

The flesh tinted cream may be used in the same

manner as the white.   The quantity to be used must rest with the person using it.

Of course, it should not be put on too thick, and it must always be put on even and smooth.   The effect of this cream upon the skin is always enhanced by thoroughly rubbing it into the skin.

Any of the white or cream preparations, either in liquid, paste, or powder form, may be tinted to any shade of flesh color by adding a small quantity of either the pure pulverized carmine or the liquid rouge.

PREPARATIONS

FOR THE COMPLEXION AND SKIN.

(*In Powder Form.*)

I fully appreciate the fact that there are a great many circumstances in connection with the use of preparations of this character that have a very large influence over the result.   It would be utterly impossible for me to enter fully into all the details of them.   I must content myself by saying that it is very essential to apply, evenly, the right quantity only, in order to avoid disappointment in their use.   If at any time, while using them, the skin becomes rough, the occasional application of one of my preparations will keep the skin in excellent condition, soft, smooth and delicate.

As the effects of different preparations vary with different people, it may be necessary to try several before the best results can be obtained.

Each one of the recipes will make a preparation that has peculiar properties of its own ; no two of them will have just the same effect; this will be demonstrated on trying them.

"THE ELITE" COMPLEXION POWDER.

This makes an exceedingly fine powder. It is a pure white, and very soft; just the powder to be highly prized by good judges of toilet powders. I have put it up for a long time for people who desired something extra nice.

Take
Pulverized Corn Starch, 12 ounces.
Pulverized Oxychlor Bismuth, 1 ounce.
Pulverized White Venetian Talc. 3 ounces.
Oil Neroli Petale, 15 drops.
Oil Sandal Wood, ½ drachm.
Oil Ceylon Cinnamon, 10 drops.
Oil Lavender Flowers, ½ drachm.

Mix the powders together well; then add the oils, (which should be previously mixed together), stirring the mixture during the time the oils are being added.

Directions.

This powder may be used upon the skin as desired; follow suggestions in special directions.

"THE MELROSE" FACE POWDER.

This recipe makes a powder that is slightly tinted; just enough to give the complexion a real youthful appearance ; it is very highly praised.

Take
Pure Precipitated Chalk, 10 ounces.
Pure Pulverized Venetian Red, 2 drachms.

Finely Pulv. Arrow Root, 2 ounces.
Oil Rose Geranium, 1 drachm
   " Cloves
   " Sweet Orange } each 20 drops.
   " Bergamot,

Prepare as follows :

Mix the Venetian Red with the Arrow Root and Chalk; then add the oils to the powder gradually; after which it must all be very thoroughly rubbed together to ensure complete incorporation. Use as desired.

It is very necessary in making Toilet Powders and powder combinations of all kinds, to be very particular to have them thoroughly and evenly mixed; they cannot be too well rubbed together or too thoroughly incorporated, to produce a fine preparation.

This should always be kept in mind whenever any of the preparations are being made.

THE PEARL POWDER FOR THE COMPLEXION.

This recipe makes another pure white preparation; it produces a most beautiful effect; it is very much admired for the smoothness and delicate hue it imparts to the skin.

Take :

Finely Pulv. Arrow Root, 11 ounces.
   " Sub. Nitrate Bismuth, ½ ounce.
Precipitated chalk, 4 ounces.
Pulv. Borax, ¼ ounce.

Oil Cloves,
" Sassafras, } each, ½ drachm.
" Winter-green)
" Cassia,   } each, 10 drops.
" Peppermint)
" Bergamot, 20 drops.

Mix the powders thoroughly; then mix the oils and gradually add them to the mixed powders; stir until completely incorporated.

The oils used must be fresh and of best quality.

Directions.

The Pearl Powder may be applied to the skin anywhere according to my special instructions. If the quality of material used in making this Powder is pure, it will make an all white powder that is equal to the best.

THE FRENCH FACE POWDER.

This recipe will make one of the most elegant face and skin Powders I ever put up. It is equal to any French preparation in the market.

This formula certainly makes an exceedingly fine Powder. It is tinted and will give to the skin a beautiful, light flesh hue, and a very fine, smooth complexion.

Take:

Finely Pulv. Oxide Zinc, 2 ounces.
  "   "   Best Starch, 8   "
  "   "   Drop Chalk, 4   "
  "   "   White Clay, 4   "
  "   "   Orris Root, 1 ounce.
  "   "   White French Chalk, 2 ounces.
  "   "   Carmine, ½ drachm.

Oil Allspice,
" Bitter Almonds, each ½ drachm.
" Sweet Orange, ⎫
" Rose Geranium, ⎬ each 1 drachm.
" Cedrat, ⎭

Prepare as follows :

Mix the Powders together thoroughly; then mix the oils together and gradually add them to the mixed powders. Keep stirring and mixing until it is all commingled.

Directions.

The French Face Powder may be used just as desired.

Apply as often as necessary, use either puff, chamois skin or soft cloth ; it may also be used on the neck and arms. The effect will be perfectly elegant. Try it.

WHITE ROSE.

COMPLEXION POWDER.

This recipe makes a pure white Powder, which may be used to the best advantage on either the face, neck or arms. It is delightfully perfumed, very fine and velvety.

It will be very much appreciated by those who desire a powder that combines the elements of simplicity and effectiveness.

Take

Finely Pulv. White Talc, ⎫
Pure Precipitate Chalk, ⎬ each, 4 ounces.
Finely Pulv. Drop Chalk, ⎭
Ottar Rose, 5 drops.

Oil Rose Geranium, 1 drachm.
" Sandal Wood, 10 drops.

Mix Powders thoroughly and add the oils gradually until they are fully divided.

Directions.

This Powder may be used as desired. It is extra nice for evening use, especially when a very pale white complexion is wanted.

ROYAL COMPLEXION POWDER.

This name might lead people to think that this Powder was designed exclusively for people of royal birth; but such is not the case ; it is used with equally as much pleasure by other people and by them declared to be a powder of *royal qualities.*

Take :

Pulv. Pure Drop Chalk, 4 ounces.
"   " Corn Starch, 12 "
Sub. Nitrate Bismuth, 1 ounce.
Oil Neroli Petale, ½ drachm.
" Lavender Flowers, 1 drachm.
" Bay Leaves, 1 drachm.
Ottar Rose, 4 drops.

Mix all the powders together; also mix the oils together, then gradually add the mixed oils to the powder, and rub them until thoroughly mixed.

Directions.

This Powder may be used as required, and be put on with puff, chamois skin or soft cloth. It has a beautiful effect when tinted to a flesh color, which can be done by the addition of carmine as suggested further back.

"NATURE'S OWN TOILET POWDER"

FOR THE COMPLEXION AND SKIN.

This formula makes a flesh-tinted powder that is very smooth and velvety; it has a fine effect upon the skin, and is a splendid powder for evening use; it gives radiance to the expression.

Take
Pulv. White Talc, 7 ounces.
Sub. Nitrate Bismuth, 1 ounce.
Pure Precipitated Chalk, 7 ounces.
Finely Pulv. Arrow Root, 1 ounce.
Pulv. Borax, 2 drachms.
Pulv. Best Carmine, 1½ drachm.
Extract Heliotrope, 2 drachms.
    "   Jasmin, 1 drachm.
Oil Bergamot, 1 drachm.

Mix the powders (which must be very fine) together; then add the extracts and oil gradually until the whole is thoroughly mixed.

Directions.

This powder may be used as required. It gives to the countenance an exceedingly bright and vivacious appearance.

BRUNETTE COMPLEXION POWDERS.

These preparations are especially adapted to Brunettes; they have a peculiar tint that is very becoming to them, suiting their complexion better than other powders.

Number 1.

Take

Pure Precipitated Chalk, 12 ounces.
Pulv. Lycopodium, 1 ounce.
    "   Best Starch, 6 ounces.
    "   French Chalk, 2 ounces.
    "   Carbonate Iron, 2½ drachms.
Oil Cloves,   ⎫
  " Lavender Flowers, ⎬ each 1 drachm.
  " Bergamot,   ⎭
  " Cedrat (Citron), ⎱ each ½ drachm.
  " Sweet Orange, ⎰

Mix the powders together; also the oils; then gradually add the oils to the powder and rub or mix together until the whole becomes completely commingled.

Directions for using.

This powder can be used just as required; it must be put on evenly all over and the effect will be gratifying. To those who desire to try this powder I would suggest that they have a small quantity put up to try.

ANOTHER BRUNETTE COMPLEXION POWDER.

Number 2.

This powder differs from the preceding one in shade of tint; and also in the effect produced. It is a most elegant preparation, soft, fine and velvety.

I can positively say that this combination has no superior. It is also delightfully perfumed·

Take

Pulv. Corn Starch, 6 ounces.
  "   Flor. Orris Root, 2 drachms.
  "   Sub. Nitrate Bismuth, 4 drachms.
  "   Pure Drop Chalk, 6 ounces.
  "   Borax, 2 drachms.
  "   Gum Gamboge, 2½ drachms.
  "   Carbonate Iron, ½ drachm.
Oil Rose Geranium, } each ½ drachm.
  "   Bay Leaves, }
  "   Sandal Wood, 1½ drachm.
  "   Lemon Grass, 20 drops.
  "   Bitter Almonds, 5 drops.

Mix the powders (which must all be very fine); next mix the oils together; then gradually add the oils to the powders; and rub together until thoroughly mixed.

Directions.

This powder can be applied as desired to the face, neck and arms.

"PEACH-BLOW POWDER"

FOR THE COMPLEXION.

This recipe, as the name implies, will make a very fine preparation; it has a beautiful tint. It is so near the natural color of the skin that it can be used without being detected. If the complexion has become sallow and of an undesirable appearance, this powder will at once give to it the appearance of blooming youth. It may be used with extraordinary good effect in completing the toilet for the evening.

Take.

Pulv. Corn Starch, 8 ounces.

" Heavy Calcined Magnesia, 3 ounces.
." White Talcum, 4 ounces.
Oil Allspice, ⎫
" Sweet Orange, ⎬ each ½ drachm.
" Sandal Wood, ⎭
" Civet, 5 drops.
Pure Carmine, 5 grains.
Aqua Ammonia, 1 drachm.

Prepare as follows :
Dissolve the carmine in the aqua ammonia, mix all the powders together; then add the solution of carmine gradually to a portion of the powder and mix it thoroughly. Then add the remainder of the powder; after this has been well mixed together, add the oils and stir until all of it is completely commingled.

When this powder is finished it should be a very' light flesh tint. It may be applied as usual.

ROUGES

FOR PRODUCING A ROSY COMPLEXION AND RUBY LIPS,

ALSO FOR BLENDING SKIN PREPARATIONS.

For rouge in the dry state use only the pure carmine.
This can be had at any of the drug stores.

Directions for using.

Put a small quantity of the carmine on a piece of chamois skin, and make it into fine powder by pressing and rubbing it between the chamois skin. This will cause the carmine to spread over the chamois skin very evenly; when this has been done it will be ready to use upon the face or lips by simply applying the chamois skin to the spot.

Do not put the rouge on too thick. It should rather be too light than too heavy; too much will over-do the matter and spoil the effect.

When a rosy complexion and red lips are desired follow the above course carefully and you will not be disappointed with the result. A very beautiful effect may be produced by using one of the white preparations for the complexion. When powder is used apply it in the usual manner; even it nicely; then apply the carmine with the chamois, just enough to bring on a beautiful flesh tint. If the white preparation is in liquid form, put it on in the usual way; allow it to dry; then carefully put on a small quantity of the carmine and blend them together. When this is done nicely it has a most charming effect.

ROUGE IN LIQUID FORM.

When a rouge is desired in this form, use the following recipe to make it, and you will have just as good rouge as can be made.

Take

> Pure Carmine, 5 grains.
> Aqua Ammonia, 1 drachm.
> Glycerine, 1 drachm.
> Rose Water, 6 drachms.

Dissolve the carmine in the ammonia; add the rose-water and glycerine; shake together and keep will corked.

Directions for using.

Apply the liquid rouge with a small soft sponge, put on only a small quantity and spread it over the surface well in order to thin it out. *Do not get it on too thick* as that would certainly spoil the effect. It should be remembered that *a little of this goes a good way.*

Some ladies love to blend their white complexion preparations on the face in this manner. The white preparation should be put on in the usual way ; nicely evened, allowed to dry, then apply a small quantity of the liquid rouge in the center of the cheek; this will produce a very handsome effect; and the blooming complexion so much admired.

MODIFIED ROUGE.

This formula makes a very handsome rouge of medium shade.

It is perhaps more properly a highly-tinted complexion powder. This powder is used alone just as it is, or in connection with pure white powder for blending. Where used as it is, it gives a very delicate rosy hue to the skin.

Take
 Pure Precipitated Chalk, 8 ounces.
  " Pulv. Oxide Zinc, 4 drachms.
  "   " Starch, 2½ ounces.
  "   " Carmine, 20 grains.
 Oil Rose Geranium, ½ drachm.
  " Lavender Flowers, ½ drachm.
  " Cloves, 20 drachms.
 Extract Musk tree, ½ drachm.

Mix the powders except the carmine together; then add the carmine to a small quantity of the other powders and rub them together ; when this has been done sufficiently to blend them, add the remainder of the powder, mix the oil and the extract together, and gradually add them to the powder; continue stirring them together until completely commingled. When completed this should be a very soft, delicate powder. Apply it as desired, either alone or by blending with white powder.

ROUGE, " LIGHT SHADE."

This recipe will make a light flesh-tinted powder. It will be very much admired for the natural hue it gives to the complexion; that is to say, it will bestow on it a color resembling the natural color of the skin, which is possessed by a person enjoying the most highly prized gift of nature, " a fresh blooming complexion."

Take

Finely Pulv. Starch 4½ ounces,
    "   " prepared Chalk ½ ounce,
Pure precipitated Chalk, 3 ounces,
    " Pulv. Carmine, 13 grains,
Oil Ylang Ylang, 10 drops,
    " Rose Geranium, 1 drachm,
Extract Musk, 1 drachm,

Mix the carmine and prepared chalk, and rub them together until finely pulverized; then add the other powders; then the oils and extract which should be previously mixed; stir together until thoroughly mixed. This powder gives very general satisfaction where a light colored rouge or tinted powder is wanted; it is very soft, smooth and fine; it gives to the skin a soft, velvety appearance.

Directions: *Use as desired.*

Ladies using any of these preparations should not neglect to study the special directions and instructions which are be found in the beginning of this book;

these will give them important information in regard to the use of the various preparations.

TOILET POWDERS.

This class of preparations are especially adapted to the drying and cooling of the skin, when overheated, or moist from excessive perspiration, and relieve irritation, itching, or soreness arising from chapping; they are also very efficacious in preventing perspiration showing upon the face and skin. They will be found especially useful during hot weather, for they act like a charm in preventing excessive perspiration and redness of the face and hands, which are always so disagreeable and often very embarrassing to ladies. They may be used several times a day if required; and materially relieve the uncomfortable feeling of irritation and soreness, frequently experienced by persons who perspire excessively during hot weather.

Do not allow these things to vex and exasperate the mind, but resort to the use of the alleviating preparations here suggested, thereby securing for yourself peace and contentment.

VIOLET POWDER.

The following recipe will make a violet toilet powder that is equal to any; it is fine, soft and velvety, richly perfumed, lasting and fragrant.

I cannot too often reiterate that all the materials used in making toilet powders should be pure and fresh; all articles in powder must be the very finest pulverized; no other grade should be tolerated.

Take

    Finely pulv. Arrow-root, 10 ounces.
    Pulv. Lycopodium,   2   "
    Finely pulv. Orris-root, 2   "
    Extract Violet, 2 drachms.
       "   Musk, $1\frac{1}{2}$ "
    Oil Ceylon-Cinnamon true, 8 drops.
     " Lavender Flower,   12 "

Prepare as follows:

Mix the powders together; then add the extracts and oils; rub them together until they are thoroughly incorporated.

These powders should always be kept in closely covered receptacles or wide-mouth bottles, well corked, to insure a highly pleasing odor.

Directions for using.

Always use puff in putting on toilet powders; when they are used upon the face they may be rubbed on, or over, with soft cloth to even them. They may also be used with charming results upon the neck and arms.

ROSE TOILET POWDER.

This recipe makes a very elegant powder; there is always something very agreeable and pleasant about it, which makes it a favorite with a great many people.

The simple and inexpensive ingredients may lead some to think that this preparation cannot be as good as those that are put up in small packages and sold in the stores. But no matter what powders, or by whom put up, there are none in the market that are superior to those made from the recipes in this book.   Try the preparations and prove it.

When you have the recipes to make the preparations, .you have what in most cases constitutes the largest part of the price paid for them.

ROSE POWDER.

Take
    Pulv. Corn-starch,   16 ounces.
    Finely Pulv. Fuller's Earth, 2   "
        "   White Talc,   2   "
    Otta Rose, 5 drops.
    Oil Rose Geranium, 1 drachm.
    Extract Musk,   ½   "
        " Jockey Club, 1   "
Prepare as follows:

Mix the powders well together; then add the extracts and oils gradually, and keep stirring until they are thoroughly commingled; use with puff as required.

WHITE ROSE,

TOILET AND NURSERY POWDERS.

This recipe makes an elegant preparation.   It is exceedingly simple and has few superiors in allaying itching and burning of the skin.   It is entirely free from all roughness, and its purity should give it a place in every nursery, where close attention to this matter is imperative.

Every mother ought to make it her special business to see that *all things used there* should be of the very purest quality.

There is no way she can know that so well as by

4 *

knowing the composition of the preparations used. The recipes will at once place the nature and character of the materials before her, and enable her to accept or reject their use for herself and children; this is the most important problem that the mother or nurse have to contend with. It certainly deserves and should have their careful consideration, and it can be handled very easily by making the preparations after the formulas in this book.

To make the White Rose powder:

Take

    Best Farina (finest powder), 16 ounces.
    Ottar Roses, 10 drops.
    Oil Ylang Ylang, 15 drops.
    " Sweet Orange, 1 drachm.

Mix the oils and gradually add them to the farina, rubbing it together until thoroughly commingled.

Directions.

This powder may be used on children very freely, as well as on the skin of grown people, as often as required.

VIOLET POWDER,

FOR THE TOILET OR NURSERY.

This recipe makes a Violet powder. It has a positive attraction that none of the ordinary powders possess, and it has properties that are peculiar to its combination. It is very smooth and velvety, and has a most beautiful effect upon the skin. It relieves sunburn, heat and chafing.

Take
Pulv. Flor. Orris root, 2 ounces.
 " Corn-starch, 12 ounces.
 " Lycopodium, 1 ounce.
Oil Neroli Petale, ½ drachm.
 " Cloves,
 " Cinnamon true, } each 15 drops.
 " Bergamot, ½ drachm.
 " Lavender Flowers, ½ drachm.

Prepare as follows:
Mix the powders, then the oils together; gradually add the oils to the powder and stir until they are well commingled.

Directions.

This powder may be used as often as required. Dust it on with puff.

VELVET TOILET POWDER.

This is a very smooth, velvety powder. It produces a most beautiful effect upon the skin, and is especially nice to use in hot weather.

Take
Finely pulv. Arrow-root, 4 ounces.
 " " Corn-starch, 4 "
 " " Oxychlor. Bismuth, 2 drachms.
 " " Orris-root, 2 ounces.
Oil Neroli Petale, 15 drops.
 " Rose Geranium, 12 drops.
 " Cloves, 4 drops.
 " Lemon, (fresh) 6 drops.

Mix the powders and add the oils gradually; the oils should be previously mixed.

This powder may be used as required; put it on with puff.

The recipes for making the toilet powders, provide for quite a quantity. A less quantity may be put up by using half or one quarter of the full amount, preserving always the proportions of the ingredients.

VARIOUS PREPARATIONS

FOR IMPROVING, PRESERVING AND BEAUTIFYING THE SKIN, ON THE HANDS, FACE, AND LIPS.

Among these will be found formulas for making preparations in all the different forms desired for this purpose. I have endeavored to have the variety large enough to enable all to suit their taste or notion on this question, so that there will be no difficulty in selecting a preparation that it will not only be a pleasure to use, but from which also the most charming results will be obtained.

In order to secure the very best effects from any of the preparations it must be remembered that only the very purest and freshest ingredients should be used in making them, and it always pays well to be very particular in applying or using any preparation of this character, for the results, to a certain extent, depend upon this. .

FRAGRANT BALM.

This recipe will make an elegant preparation to use upon the skin. There is none superior or pleasanter to use. It allays irritation, itching, smarting, and cures chapped and rough skin at once. It imparts to the skin a brilliant transparency which is pleasing and very much admired.

Take

Best Quince Seed, ½ ounce.
Pure Water, 7 ounces.
Pure Glycerine, 1½ ounce.
Alcohol, 4½ ounces.
Salicylic Acid, 6 grains.
Pure Carbolic Acid, 10 grains.
Oil Bay Leaves, 10 drops.
   "   Cloves, 5 drops.
   "   Sweet Orange, 10 drops.
   "   Winter-green, 8   "
   " Ottar-Rose, 2 drops.

Prepare as follows :

Dissolve the Salicylic acid in the alcohol; then add the oils. Add the carbolic acid to the glycerine, shake together, and set these two mixtures to one side; then digest the quince seed in the water for 24 hours; have it standing in a moderately warm place ; then strain it through cloth, using some pressure of the hand if necessary, to bring it through the strainer. When this has been done nicely, add all together, shake well, and it is ready to use. Keep in bottle well corked.

Directions for using.

The best time to apply this preparation is at night before retiring. This holds good in relation to any preparation of this character, as it can then remain on all night without being disturbed.

Of course it may be applied through the day several times if necessary. If a *small quantity* is put on the hands right after washing them, it will have a splendid effect. It should be rubbed on quick and hard in order to get it into the pores of the skin well. If your skin is rough or badly chapped, do not fail to try this. It is a conceded fact that this preparation is not excelled by any for roughness of the skin. It is free from the greasy and sticky features that are so objectionable in a great many preparations.

RUBY CREAM.

FOR THE LIPS AND HANDS.

This preparation will cure cracked and chapped lips or hands. It is almost a specific for cold sores.

Take

Rose Cosmoline, 3 ounces.
Pulv. Camphor, 5 grains.
Balsam Peru, 1½ drachms.
Pulv. Carmine, 8 grains.
Oil Cinnamon Tree, 5 drops.
" Anise Seed, 6 drops.

The Carmine should be in a very fine powder ; add it to the cosmoline, then add all the other ingredients. When completed it will be a very fine creamy-like salve, of a handsome color and agreeable odor.

Directions for using.

For cracked or chapped lips, apply at night before retiring; use the finger to put it on. It may be applied also through the day. Use it in the same way for cold sores. For chapped, cracked or rough hands it should be well rubbed on after bathing ; also apply and rub it on the hands just before retiring. It is a good plan to put on a pair of old gloves, to prevent soiling the linen, and to keep it well on the hands. It will soften the skin and improve the appearance of the hands very much. What is more admired than a beautiful pair of hands—and what is more unsightly than hands which are rough, coarse, chapped, swollen and red, especially if these are ladies' hands? The use of this cream occasionally will make the hands soft and white, and the skin smooth and velvety.

GLYCERINE BALM FOR THE SKIN.

This recipe will make a preparation different from most others. It is richly perfumed, and has other desirable features which makes it a very pleasant preparation to use.

Take
 Pure White Starch, pulv., ½ ounce.
 Water,
 Pure Glycerine, each 1 ounce
 Bay Rum, 2 drachms.
 Oil Bergamot. 8 drops.
  " Rose Geranium. 2 drops.
 Extract Jockey Club, 2 drachms.
  " Cochineal Comp. ½ drachm.

Mix the glycerine, water and starch; place over a *gentle* fire; heat very slowly; keep stirring it all the time; this must be done to prevent burning. When it becomes creamy and pasty, take it from the fire; allow it to become nearly cold, then stir in the extract cochineal, Jockey Club, bay rum and oils of bergamot and geranium. It is necessary to be very particular in making this preparation; it must not be left on the fire for an instant after it is warm without being stirred; for just as sure as it is, it will certainly burn and be spoiled.

If the instructions are followed a beautiful preparation will result.

Directions for Using.

The best effect is produced by applying to the skin just after bathing and before drying it; rub the balm over the surface, then wipe dry with a towel.

This may be done as often as required. It can also be used on the dry skin.

COLD CREAM.

This is a preparation that has been used by nearly everybody, and all know something about it. The following recipe will make a cold cream which is not excelled by any; it is pleasantly perfumed; will not become rancid, as too many do; above all, it is a very efficacious preparation, and soothing and healing to the skin:

Take

 Spermaceti, ½ ounce.
 White Wax, ½ ounce.
 Rose Cosmoline, 1 ounce.
 Oil Sweet Almonds, 4 ounces.
 Rose Water, 3 ounces.
 Pulv. Borax, 40 grains.
 Oil Rose Geranium, 20 drops.
  " Patchouly 6 drops.
  " Ylang Ylang, 6 drops.

Prepare as Follows :

Melt the spermaceti, wax and cosmoline, over a little fire. Dissolve the borax in the rose water, and gradually add the solution to the almond oil. It should be. agitated continually while adding it, the harder the better. After the oil, borax and water have become thoroughly incorporated and the mixture has a white, creamy or milky appearance; and while the melted wax, sperm and cosmoline are still warm, add the two mixtures together, gradually stirring it all the time. It should be kept moderately warm. Then take off fire and keep stirring the whole until nearly cold, when the oils of the rose, geranium, patchouly and ylang ylang should be added and the mixture again be stirred very thoroughly for a few minutes. It should be, when complete, of a very rich, creamy appearance, and of a nice smooth consistence. When properly prepared this recipe will make an elegant cold cream.

Directions.

Apply to the parts affected several times a day, and just before retiring at night; it may be used for all kinds of skin difficulties.

GOLDEN CREAM.

This recipe makes a preparation that is a specific for roughness, inflammation, soreness, chafing, and irritation of the skin.

There is a similarity between this and cold cream. Yet there is a vast difference in their character when completed.

. Take

Oil Sweet Almonds, 1½ ounce.
Pure Yellow Bees-wax, 2 drachms.
Spermaceti, ½ ounce.
Rose-water, 2 drachms.

Rose Cosmoline, 1 ounce.
Oil Cinnamon-true, 4 drops.
" Bitter Almonds, 2 "
Pulv. Winter-green, 10 "
" Borax, 20 grains.

Prepare as follows :

Place the Bees-wax and spermaceti in a suitable dish ; place this over a gentle fire ; when they are nearly melted add the cosmoline ; allow them all to melt and unite ; this can be hastened by stirring it ; then take off from fire ; dissolve the borax in the rose-water and add it to the oil of sweet almonds, stirring it constantly while adding ; after it has been well mixed add the mixture to the melted wax, sperm, and cosmoline, very slowly ; stir briskly while it is being added ; when they are all thoroughly incorporated and nearly cold add the other oils ; mix them in well. Do not allow the melted wax, sperm, and cosmoline to get too cold and stiff before adding the rose-water, almond oil and borax mixture. If you do it will become hard and lumpy, which will necessitate its being placed over the fire just long enough to warm it through ; then stir briskly for a short time, this will generally bring it out all right.

When the Golden Cream is prepared properly, it makes a most beautiful preparation. It will keep any length of time.

Directions for using.

Apply at night before retiring. It may also be applied through the day.

This cream may be used upon the most delicate skin with the most charming results. For softening and beautifying the skin, it will be found in advance of all others.

COMEDONE CREAM.

This formula will make a preparation that is not excelled by any for removing *blackheads pimples and blemishes* of all kinds from the skin; it is of the highest advantage as an external application in connection with a blood purifier in eruptions on the skin of whatever character. It will relieve and often effect a cure of the intense itching experienced by those having some form of the various skin diseases.

I can safely say to those afflicted, it can do no harm, and may do good in your case, as it has in others ; give it a trial.

Take

 Washed Sulphur, 1 ounce.

 Pulv. White Clay, 6 drachms.

 Pure Glycerine, 6   "

 Acetic Acid, 4 drachms.

 Oil Sandal Wood, ½ drachm.

  " Patchouly, 10 drops.

  " Bergamot, 30   "

Mix the clay and sulphur with the glycerine and acetic acid; then add the oils and rub all together very thoroughly.

Directions for using.

This should be applied at night with a fine moistened sponge ; put it on to the affected parts; leave on over night, and wash off in the morning.

If this treatment is persisted in, it rarely fails to

effect a cure of the most obstinate cases. It should be put on thick enough to form a light coating, but not too heavy.

DERMAL CREAM.

FOR CHAPPED HANDS, LIPS OR FACE.

The following recipe will make a preparation that gives good results when most things fail.

Take
    Rose Cosmoline, 2 ounces.
    Pure Carbolic Acid, 10 grains.
    Tincture Benzoin, plain, 2 drachms.
    Oil Cade, ½ drachms.
    " Sassafras, 15 drops.
    " Lemon, *fresh*, 10 drops.

Prepare as follows:

Mix all the ingredients well together; to insure thorough mixing, it should be rubbed together in a mortar or on a pill tile.

Directions for using.

Apply to the parts affected.

If used upon the hands, it should be applied after washing them; also before retiring at night.

After it has been applied and thoroughly rubbed in, put on a pair of old thread gloves over night.

THE J. A. B. CREAM FROTH.

FOR RENDERING THE SKIN SOFT, SMOOTH AND TRANSPARENT.

This recipe will make a preparation which imparts a beautiful transparency to the skin. It leaves it smooth and velvety. It is a splendid preparation for roughness of the skin. I have sold it for a long time with the utmost satisfaction.

After it is used a short time its merits will be appreciated.

Take

Pure Glycerine, 2 ounces.
Oil Sweet Almonds, 2 ounces.
Liquor Potassa, 2 drachms.
Rose Water, 2 ounces.
Extract Musk (best), 1 drachm.
Oil Winter-green, 15 drops.
" Cloves, 10 drops.
" Sassafras, 5 drops.
" Neroli Petale, 5 drops.

Prepare as follows:

Add the liquor potassa to the oil almonds; shake it thoroughly for a short time, then add the glycerine and other oils; then give the mixture a lengthy shaking in order to thoroughly mix it; then add the extract musk and rose water and shake once more.

Directions for using.

It should always be well shaken before it is used.

It may be applied several times a day, but it is best to use it just before retiring, as being on over night gives it a chance to take a hold.

The surface of the skin should be well covered with it, and it should be rubbed on hard in order to get it into the pores; in the morning it should be washed off and the skin rubbed gently with a soft towel.

"EXCELSIOR BALM."

FOR MAKING THE HANDS SOFT AND SMOOTH.

It is surprising how this preparation will preserve

the hands and keep them free from all roughness. It is also just the thing needed by people who have their hands in and out of the water a great deal; it will positively keep them in fine condition. I speak with the full knowledge of its merits, for I have seen it used a number of years with gratifying results.

Take
>Rose Water, 1 ounce.
>Pure Glycerine, 3 ounces.
>Pulv. Borax, 2 drachms.
>Bay Rum, 5 ounces.
>Pure Carbolic Acid, 20 grains.
>Extract Heliotrope, 1½ drachm.
>   " Vanilla, pure, 1½ drachm.
>Oil Sandal Wood, 10 drops.

Dissolve the borax in the glycerine by agitating it; then add bay rum, rose water, carbolic acid, extracts and oil.

Directions for using.

Keep the excelsior balm convenient to where you are in the habit of bathing the hands; after washing and before drying them pour a small quantity of it into the palm of the hand and rub it over the hands thoroughly; then dry carefully with towel. It is very necessary they should be completely dried after using the Balm and before exposing them to the weather. It may also be put on at night before retiring.

"CARBOLIZED GLYCERINE AND ROSE WATER."

This preparation really needs no introduction to a great many people, for it has been used by them for a long time and its merits as a preparation for the preservation and improvement of the skin are well known. But to those that have not used the combination I would suggest that they give it a trial and thus test its excellence.

Take
    Pure Glycerine,
    Rose Water,
    Alcohol, each 1 ounce.
    Pure Carbolic Acid, 25 grains.
    Extract Heliotrope, 1½ drachm.
    "   Jockey Club, 1½ drachm.

Mix the glycerine and carbolic acid together; then add the alcohol and rose water, shake well, add the extracts; then shake all together.

Directions for using.

Apply with finger lightly to parts affected; when used upon the hands apply after washing them, and at night before retiring, rub it on very thoroughly; then cover the hands with old thread gloves.

This treatment will relieve and cure very bad cases of chapped or cracked skin on the hands.

If it should smart too much reduce with a small amount of water.

"HAND POWDER."

COMPOUND ALMOND POWDER, FOR MAKING THE HANDS WHITE, SOFT, AND SMOOTH.

This recipe will make a preparation that has the property of making the hands all that could be desired.

Take

    Fine Almond Meal, 4 ounces.

    Pulv. Borax, 6 drachms.

       "   Orris-root, 2 ounces.

       "   Pumice Stone, 6 drachms.

    Oil Bitter Almonds, 8 drops.

       " Sassafras, 10 drops.

Mix the powders thoroughly and add the oils; stir together till they are well mixed.

Directions for using.

This powder may be used very freely on the hands just after bathing them; while they are still wet rub on long enough to dry them; then brush surplus powder off. Or it may be used as a soap powder, to wash the hands; rubbing real hard with it, then rinse off and dry them with towel. This powder may also be used to good advantage on the neck and arms.

"COMPOUND ORRIS POWDER."

This is another preparation used very satisfactorily for whitening and softening the hands, and for making the skin soft and transparent. Its use will improve and beautify the hands and complexion.

In some respects it is superior to the Compound Almond Powder, although they are both excellent combinations and will no doubt be very much liked when their merits become known.

Take

    Pulv. Flor Orris-root, 8 ounces.

       "   Bicarbonate Soda, 1 ounce.

       "   Corn Meal, 3 ounces.

Ess. Oil Bitter Almonds, 8 drops.
"   Rose Geranium, 20 drops.
"   Nutmegs, 20 drops.

Mix the powders; then gradually add the oils, and mix all thoroughly together.

These hand powders should be kept in wide bottles, well corked.

Directions for using.

Keep it convenient to where the hands are washed; before drying take enough of the powder in the hands to rub it all over them thoroughly. Keep on rubbing till the water has been taken up and the hands are dry ; then rinse them off with tepid water, after which dry them with a soft towel.

This powder can also be used upon the face, neck and arms, in same way as above, or it may be put on in a dry state and the skin well rubbed with it.

CHAFING POWDER.

This preparation will prevent and cure chafing and excessive perspiration. There are very few things that give more trouble than these to many persons.

It is also an excellent toilet powder, and has a soothing effect upon the skin, which makes it very agreeable to use.

Take
Pulv. White Talcum, 6 ounces.
"   Lycopodium, 1 ounce.
"   Starch, 2 ounces.
Oil Sweet Orange, $\frac{1}{2}$ drachm.
" Rose Geranium, $\frac{1}{2}$ drachm.
5

" Lavender Flowers, 15 drops.
" Peppermint, 5 drops.
" Sassafras, 3 drops.

Mix the powders together; then add the oils and rub them together until they are thoroughly mixed.

Directions for using.

Apply powder with puff. Dust it on freely to the parts affected. To prevent chafing and soreness, simply dust this powder on with puff to the different parts. This will effectually prevent it. It is also very cooling to the overheated skin. This may be relieved by dusting the powder over the surface. It will frequently allay irritation and itching of the skin by dusting it on to the affected parts.

LOTIONS.

Under this head will be found lotions of various kinds, with full instructions for their uses and purposes. The recipes for making the different preparations are all thoroughly reliable, and will produce effects which are not to be surpassed.

THE RHODA CREAM LOTION,

FOR SOFTENING, WHITENING, AND BEAUTIFYING THE SKIN.

This recipe makes a preparation which is truly an elegant one to use, and the effects will please.

Take

Tincture Benzoin, plain,
Tincture Myrrh, each 25 drops.

Glycerine, *pure*, 2 ounces.
Pulv. Borax, 2 drachms.
Extract Heliotrope, 2 drachms.
      " White Rose, 2 drachms.
Plain Water, 14 ounces.

Dissolve the borax in the glycerine; add the water to it; then slowly drop in the benzoin and myrrh, (they should be mixed beforehand,) stirring it all the time; next add the extracts and shake well together. This should be put into a pint bottle and kept well corked.

Directions.

Apply to the skin with a fine soft sponge, night and morning; let it dry on and remain there over night; and when it is applied in the morning it may be washed off during the day.

A small quantity of this lotion added to the bath water will impart to it a very agreeable odor, and render the skin soft and fragrant.

SHAVING LOTION,

FOR GENTLEMEN TO USE AFTER SHAVING, TO PREVENT THE FACE CHAPPING, AND TO CLEAR UP THE SKIN.

This recipe makes a very superior preparation for the face after shaving; it will positively prevent its becoming sore. It imparts a very cooling, soothing sensation to the tender skin, and is just the thing to use during warm weather.

Take
  Rose Water, 2 ounces.
  Pure Alcohol, 4 ounces.
  Pure Glycerine, 1 ounce.
  Pulv. Borax, 2 drachms.
  Comp. Spirits Lavender, 1 drachm.
  Extract Jockey Club. } Each 2 drachms.
  Extract Ylang Ylang. }
  Pure Water, 8 ounces.

Dissolve the borax in the glycerine; add the rose water, alcohol and other ingredients; shake well together.

Directions.

Apply just the same as bay rum.

THE "RHODA" TOILET LOTION.

For rendering the skin soft, smooth and transparent; for allaying smarting, burning and itching of the skin; to relieve the pain and smarting of sunburns; to cure roughness of the skin, resulting from exposure or from the use of impure soaps; to relieve and cure Salt Rheum. It may also be used for any of the various skin diseases with benefit. Apply it to the skin or surface of the body.

Take
  Oil Sweet Almonds, 1½ ounce.
  Very best Glycerine, 2½ ounces.
  Alcohol, 4 ounces.
  Ess. Oil Bitter Almonds, 12 drops.
  Oil Cinnamon Tree, 5 drops.
  Oil Sweet Orange, 1 drachm.
  Extract Musk, 1 drachm.

Mix the glycerine with the oil of sweet almonds;

shake together very thoroughly until it becomes creamy ; then add the other oils and extract musk, and give it a good shaking : then add the alcohol and shake once more ; it will then be ready for use.

Directions for using.

Shake well; apply the lotion to the parts affected, with either the fingers or soft piece of cloth; rub it on hard in order to get it into the pores of the skin. It should be applied two or three times a day and before retiring at night. When used upon the hands it should be applied right after washing them, and before drying them pour a small quantity in palm of the hand and rub over the hands while they are still moist. Keep rubbing until the hands are nearly dry, then wipe them thoroughly with a dry towel. If necessary, apply to the hands at night before retiring, without washing them ; then slip on a pair of old gloves (thread is the best); this will prevent soiling the linen. For use upon the skin anywhere else, apply several times a day ; also at night ; rub it in well each time.

THE CREAM LOTION,

FOR ALLAYING IRRITATION, REDNESS AND ROUGHNESS OF THE HANDS, FACE, AND OF THE SURFACE OF THE SKIN GENERALLY.

The following recipe is one I have used a number of years in making this lotion. It will make an extra fine and efficacious preparation, containing as it does the healing and soothing properties of glycerine and pure olive oil, combined in such a manner that the very best effects are obtained from it.

It is very pleasantly perfumed. It does not **excite** or inflame the skin, as some lotions do, but soothes **and** allays all inflammation and irritation.

It is also a very superior remedy for removing **tan,** sunburn, or discolorations from the skin. It can be used anywhere that a soothing and healing lotion is required, with the very best results.

Take

    Purest fresh Olive Oil, ½ ounce.
       "   " Glycerine, 1½ ounce.
       "   " Alcohol, 2 ounces.
    Liquor Potassa, 10 drachms.
    Oil Cloves, 10 drops.
    " Lavender Flowers, 20 drops.
    " Patchouly, 8 drops.
    " Sandal Wood · 15 "

Prepare as follows :

Add the liquor potassa to the olive oil and shake them thoroughly; then add the glycerine, and continue shaking until the mixture becomes very milky and creamy ; then add the other oils, and again shake well ; then add the alcohol. Complete by giving it a brisk shaking up.

Directions for using.

Always shake the lotion well before using it. It should be applied to the parts affected with the hand or finger; rub it on thoroughly, except when used upon the face; then it should be applied with a soft cloth and allowed to dry on ; it may be rubbed in very gently. The best time to apply it to the face is before retiring. Let it remain on all night and wash it off in the morning.

THE COMPLEXION LOTION.

FOR REMOVING BLEMISHES FROM THE FACE.

This preparation produces wonderful effects on some skins ; it frequently has cleared up a badly blemished complexion when all other things have failed. It has a very agreeable odor ; it is nice to use in hot weather, as it imparts a very fresh and agreeable odor to the skin, and has a cooling effect upon it. It is an excellent preparation for relieving sunburn, and other smarting and burning conditions of the skin.

Take

Pulv. Muriate Ammonia, 1 drachm.
" Sulphite Sodium, 2 drachms.
" Borax, 2 drachms.
Pure Glycerine, 1 ounce.
Cologne Water, 2 ounces.
Tinct. Tolu, 1 drachm.
Plain Water, 13 ounces.

Dissolve the borax, ammonia, and soda in the water ; add the glycerine, cologne water, and tincture tolu.

Directions for using.

Apply to the face several times a day and at night ; allow it to dry on each time. Use a sponge or soft cloth in putting it on.

FRECKLES ON THE SKIN.

There is probably nothing more annoying, or which causes more chagrin than those troublesome little spots upon the face and neck commonly called freckles. Some people who happen to be affected with them imagine that impertinent observers have their eyes riveted upon these disfigurements, although generally there is nothing in it but imagination. To assist these unfortunate people, I will place here a few recipes, through which I hope to give relief to those who feel that freckles are a blemish. With the preparations made after these recipes the skin can be made very clear and the complexion materially improved. There are many who will appreciate these recipes very much.

FRECKLE ERADICATOR.

Take
Sulpho. Carbolate Zinc, 1 drachm.
Rose Water, 3½ ounces.
Pure Glycerine, ½ ounce.
Extract Jockey Club, 1 drachm.
Dissolve the sulpho. carbolate zinc in the rose water; add the glycerine and extract; then shake all well together.

Directions.

Apply to the parts affected night and morning, with a soft, small sponge.

This treatment must often be persisted in a long time; so don't get easily discouraged, and give up; but persevere until you have tried it a sufficient time. If it then fails, try the following preparation.

THE OCCIDENT FRECKLE LOTION.

This recipe makes one of the very best preparations for the speedy cure and removal of tan and freckles on the skin.

The propriety of having the corrosive sublimate in the preparation might be questioned by some as a harsh remedy. But the amount used is so small that there can no possible danger arise from it. When it is properly used there is nothing to compare with it in satisfactory results, without in any way producing ill effects.

If those afflicted with freckles are desirous of getting rid of them, I would advise them to begin early the use of this preparation.

Take
    Tincture Benzoin plain, 10 drops.
    Corrosive Sublimate, 4 grains.
    Pure Glycerine, 2 drachms.
    Peppermint Water, 1 ounce.
    Pure Drop Chalk, ½ ounce.
    Orange Flower Water, 1½ ounce.
    Plain Water, 6 ounce.
    Alcohol, 1 ounce.

Dissolve the corrosive sublimate in the alcohol; then add the water and other ingredients; the tincture benzoin should be put in last.

The effects of this lotion are truly wonderful; removing all blemishes and clearing the skin in a most remarkable manner.

This proportion should be marked POISON on account of containing the corrosive sublimate.

Directions for the using the Occident Lotion :—Apply to the affected parts lightly with soft sponge or cloth, night and morning; allow it to dry on. After using this lotion for a time, the skin will show signs of becoming rough and peeling off; the use of the lotion should then be discontinued until the old skin comes off and new is formed. If the blemishes, tan, pimples and freckles still are present use the lotion a second time:

follow the treatment just the same as many times as may be necessary to produce the desired effect; always leave off applying it when the skin becomes rough and begins to peal off, if this preparation is used occasionally it will keep the skin in a clear condition and entirely free from these objectionable blemishes.

It must however be remembered that the Occident Lotion is not designed to be used regularly; it will make the face sore if used too long; it is only intended to be used for a short period.

THE FRECKLE LOTION.

This recipe will makes a preparation for removing freckles and tan which is very much milder than the preceding lotion. It is just the thing for people to use who have a very tender skin. It is a very efficacious remedy, and in a great many cases serves the purpose better than the more powerful Occident Lotion. Of course there are cases that require an extra strong remedy. But where a milder one will serve the purpose use the following.

Take

Pure Gran. Muriate Ammonia, 3 drachms.
"   "   Sulphate Zinc, 20 grains.
"   Glycerine, 1 ounce.
Extract Jockey Club, 2 drachms.
Pure Water, 14 ounces.

Dissolve the ammoniac and zinc in the water; add the glycerine and jockey club; shake well together.

Directions for using:—This lotion may be applied with a small sponge or soft cloth several times through the day and at night before retiring it should be applied very thoroughly. Allowing it to dry on the skin each time after putting on, will enhance its effects.

PIMPLE LOTION.

This recipe makes a preparation that will remove those disagreeable blotches that disfigure the faces of some people and which are a source of mortification to them. There are few things which are more displeasing to the eye than to see a young lady or gentleman, with the face and forehead all covered with ugly looking blotches, red pimples, and little pustules. It generally embarrasses the unfortunate person greatly.

The following preparations will usually afford relief when used in connection with some good constitutional treatment. There is nothing that serves the purpose better than one of the blood purifiers, for which recipes are to be found in this book; when the applications fail to produce the desired results, or during their use, take regularly some good constitutional medicine.

The pimple lotion is made as follows:

Take
  Iodide Potassa, 3 drachms.
  Camphor Water, 3 ounces.
  Cologne   "   ½   "
  Peppermint "   1   "
  Rose   "   1½ "
  Spirits Lavender Comp., 1 drachm.

Dissolve the iodide potassa in the rose water; add the peppermint water, camphor water, cologne water and spirits lavender ; shake well together.

Directions.—Apply with soft sponge or cloth three or four times a day and at night before retiring; allow it to dry on after each application.

LOTION,

FOR TREATING PRICKLY HEAT.

The following recipe makes a preparation which I have found generally efficacious in relieving and curing this most distressing complaint. I have seen extra good results from its use in some very severe cases.

Take

Pure Alcohol, 1 ounce.
" Glycerine, 1 ounce.
Pulv. Camphor, 10 grains.
Pure Carbolic Acid, 10 grains.
Peppermint Water, 2 ounces.
Extract Jockey Club, ½ drachm.

Dissolve the camphor in the alcohol; add the carbolic acid and glycerine; then shake well, and add the peppermint water and extract jockey club; shake all together.

Directions for using :—This lotion should be applied slightly to the affected parts several times a day, varying according to the severity and condition of the complaint.

LOTION,

OF HONEY AND BORAX.

For roughness of the skin, this preparation is very

much admired by some people. It is also an excellent remedy for tan and sunburn; it is a very simple and yet effective combination. I have prepared it many times for those who found it very beneficial.

It works like a charm in relieving and curing some cases of sore mouth; it is perfectly harmless; it can therefore be used anywhere on any kind of abrasions.

Take

Pure Strained Honey, 1½ ounce.
Pulv. Borax, 1 ounce.
Pure Glycerine, 1½ ounce.
Ext. White Rose, 2 drachms.
Pure Water, 12 ounces.

Dissolve the borax in the honey; then add the glycerine; shake well together; then add the ext. white rose and water; then shake well together.

Directions for using.—When this lotion is used for sore mouth, the latter must be thoroughly rinsed and washed with it. When used, upon the surface for roughness, irritation, or any other purpose, it may be applied in the most convenient way several times a day and before retiring at night. It also answers for a great many purposes, especially when a soothing, healing application is wanted.

PART II.

PREPARATIONS FOR THE TEETH.

IT is said that " cleanliness is next to godliness." It certainly behooves us to give heed to this golden proverb.

It is a conceded fact that good health depends upon cleanliness, and where is this necessity more apparent than in the mouth? Therefore everybody should use some good dentrifrice to keep the teeth and mouth in a clean condition, preserve and beautify the teeth, cleanse and sweeten the mouth and breath, and promote health, happiness and beauty.

I have appended a number of recipes for making preparations for the teeth, which will compare with any made, and surpass the majority of them.

This will enable everybody to select a preparation for the teeth in either the powder, liquid or paste form. All of the formulas will make meritorious preparations; they will surely prove very satisfactory on being used.

As tastes differ so much in relation to the use of a preparation of this character, it will be necessary for each person to select the particular form and character of the dentifrice, from the large number of recipes I have introduced in this treatise.

Directions and instructions for using Dentifrices :— Tooth powders cannot be prescribed daily as a strict rule. Conditions vary greatly; it must therefore be left to the judgment of each individual, just how often to use the powder. In some cases every day, in others from one to four or five times a week is sufficient.

In using tooth powders always moisten the brush thoroughly in pure water; then put on some of the powder and apply to the teeth and gums in such quantity as may be necessary to thoroughly cleanse them.

It is comparatively an easy matter to keep the teeth in a nice condition, and to have them look white and clean. There is no way this can be done better than by the use of the preparations for the teeth to be made from the recipes in this book. As the teeth of different persons require such different treatment, it is a very difficult matter to lay down a set of rules that will be suitable for all. Therefore the character of the preparations used for their preservation and for improving and beautifying them must necessarily vary greatly. Each person must, to a certain extent, be his own doctor, in selecting and using a dentifrice. Every person's taste has a very large influence in deciding what kind of a preparation to employ. Use those preparations that seem to be the best adapted to each individual case. If it is a powder, it should be used by first moistening the tooth brush in pure water; then put on the brush some of the powder and thoroughly brush the teeth; give to the brush an up and down motion over the teeth. After repeating this several times, change the operation by moving the brush back and forth over the teeth. When this has been done (not harshly but gently) several times, rinse the mouth with pure water.

In most instances it is proper to clean the teeth often, but do not brush too hard, and use a moderately soft brush.

The care of the teeth should be carefully attended to. The proper use of a good dentifrice, such as can be made from the recipes following, will preserve the teeth to old age. It only requires a little time to see to them, and yet how many people allow them to become decayed, and finally have to lose them, whereas, if they had given them proper attention and care they would have had their natural teeth in a healthy condition for a good many years.

The directions and instructions for using tooth preparations in liquid and paste forms will be found under the recipes for making them.

Tooth powder should be kept in bottles tightly corked in order to preserve their aroma. When the quantity of powder is small, this may seem unnecessary; but it is decidedly better to keep it tightly covered in either a box or bottle.

THE UNEXCELLED TOOTH POWDER.

This recipe will make a tooth powder that has no superior for cleansing, preserving and beautifying the teeth, or for hardening the gums, and perfuming the breath. It is very much admired by people who have tried its wonderful merits. It will completely arrest the progress of decay in the teeth and strengthen the gums when they are tender.

Take

Pulv. Drop Chalk,
   "   Precipitated Chalk, } each 4 ounces.
   "   Cuttle Bone, 1½ ounce.
Heavy Calcined Magnesia, ½ ounce.

Pulv. Borax, ½ drachm.
"   Carmine, 20 grains.
"   Myrrh, ½ ounce.
"   Orris-Root, 2 ounces.
"   White Castile Soap, 3 ounces.
Oil Cinnamon, ½ drachm.
"   Anise, ½ drachm.
"   Cloves, ½ drachm.
"   Wintergreen, ½ drachm.
"   Peppermint, ½ drachm.

The powdered ingredients must be in the finest powder; they should all be mixed together with the exception of the carmine; this should be added to a small part of the mixed powder, and fully incorporated; then add the remainder of the powder and mix all together until the carmine is thoroughly commingled; then add the oils gradually.

The powder should be stirred well during the time the oils are being added.

Use by moistening the tooth brush in pure water; then put on some of the powder and thoroughly cleanse the teeth with it.

AROMATIC TOOTH POWDER.

This is an exceedingly fine powder for the teeth and gums; it will be noticed that it is somewhat different from the general run of tooth powders. As a preserver and beautifier of the teeth, this powder stands at the head of all aromatic tooth preparations. By its aromatic and odorizing influences it renders the mouth sweet and gives to the breath a delightfully refreshing perfume, making it a pleasure to your associates. What is more offensive and disagreeable than a bad breath? And it is generally caused by the teeth being in a bad condition through negligence.

The use of this preparation will soon overcome that; for it will preserve the teeth, arrest decay, and harden the gums.

Take

Pulv. Cinnamon (best quality).
" Jamaica Ginger, } each ½ ounce.
" Cloves,
" Nutmegs,
" Gum Myrrh, } each 2 drachms.
" Cardamon Seeds,
" Pure Drop Chalk, } each 6 ounces.
" Flor Orris Root,
" White Sugar, 4 ounces.
" White Castle Soap, 2 ounces.
Oil Peppermint, 20 drops.
" Anise Seed, ½ drachm.

The powdered ingredients must be the finest pulverized; mix them together very thoroughly; then add the oils gradually, and mix all together until they are commingled.

Directions for using.—This powder should be used with a medium brush, not too hard, and yet not too soft; moisten it well with pure water; then put on a small amount of powder and apply to the teeth. Use it every one, two or three days, as may be necessary to keep the teeth and gums in a good healthy condition.

———

THE "WHITE" TOOTH POWDER.

This recipe makes a tooth powder equal to any all white tooth powder made. It is a recipe that I have used for a great many years for making a white tooth powder, and it became very popular under a name that was given to it, which, however, did not disclose the originator. I do positively assert that this preparation will give excellent satisfaction. It has been used for years by thousands of people and prescribed by prominent dentists, to all of whom it gave very satisfactory results. It can be made for less than it takes to buy it when prepared and sold in small bottles. If you wish a first-class all white tooth powder do not hesitate to have this recipe put up. It will justify my praise.

Take
Pure Precipitated Chalk, 8 ounces.
" Pulv. White Castile Soap, 2 ounces.
" " White Sugar, 2 ounces.
" " Bicarbonate Soda, ½ ounce.
Oil Wintergreen, 2 drachms.

Mix the Powder very thoroughly; then gradually add the oil and mix still more to insure complete commingling.

Directions.—This powder may be used just as often as desired. It will preserve, improve and beautify the teeth, harden the gums, perfume the breath, and keep the mouth sweet.

PEARL TOOTH POWDER.

This recipe also makes an extra dentifrice for preserving the teeth and hardening the gums.

Take
Pulv. Drop Chalk, 12 ounces.

Pulv. White Sugar, 4 ounces.
    "   Flor Orris-root, 2 ounces.
    "   White Castile Soap, 2 ounces.
    "   Gum Myrrh, 2 drachms.
    "   Peruvian Bark, 2 drachms.
Salicylic Acid, 20 grains.
Oil Wintergreen, 4 drachms.

Directions.—Mix the powders all together; then add the oil gradually; keep stirring until it is all very thoroughly mixed.

This is a very superior powder for the teeth; it may be used just as required.

THE "FRANKLIN" TOOTH POWDER.

Some people that have used this powder think very highly of it. It has some features which are not found in a great many tooth powders; it has proved itself to have properties for preserving, improving and beautifying the teeth that are very much admired by those who have used it.

Take
Pulv. Flor Orris-root, 8 ounces.
    "   White Sugar, 5 ounces.
    "   Drop Chalk, 6 ounces.
    "   White Castile Soap, 2 ounces.
    "   Cochineal, 2 drachms.
    "   Pure Cream Tartar, ½ ounce.
Oil Peppermint, 20 drops.
    "   Wintergreen,
    "   Anise, each 1 drachm.

Mix the powders all together; the cochineal must be very finely pulverized; mix the oils together and add them to a small quantity of the powder and mix thoroughly; then add the remainder of the powder and stir together until all are well mixed.

This powder may be used just as required.

WHITE ROSE TOOTH POWDER.

This dentifrice has some very desirable features and can be classed among the very best. It will impart a delightful taste to the mouth; remove all tartar and impurities from the teeth and completely arrest the progress of decay; it will also whiten and beautify them and strengthen and harden the gums.

Take
    Pure Precipitated Chalk, 7 ounces.
    Pulv. Sugar of Milk, 3 ounces.
      "   Bicarbonate Soda, ½ ounce.
      "   Cuttle Bone, 2 ounces.
      "   White Castile Soap, 2 ounces.
    Otta of Roses, 4 drops.
    Oil Rose Geranium, 25 drops.
      "   Sassafras, ½ drachm.

Mix the powders thoroughly; add the oils gradually and rub together until they are fully commingled.

This elegant powder may be used just as required. See Directions and Instructions.

Making the different tooth powders will not require any great amount of experience. Anybody will be able to do it with the plain instructions for each of the recipes. It is only necessary to buy the materials wanted; most generally the different powders will be put together by the druggist of whom you buy them; and so also will the different oils. If convenient use a fine sieve in mixing them according to the instructions under each recipe; it can be done with a small amount of labor. Place a clean sheet of paper upon the table; place the sieve on it; put the powder into the sieve and run it through; then add the oils to the powder; stir it with a long knife while the oil is being added; then run through the sieve a sufficient number of times to thoroughly mix everything together. This process carried out will make tooth powder as well as it can be made by any practical person, who might perhaps manipulate the components a little differently, but after all would produce no better combination.

ELEGANT SAPONACEOUS TOOTH POWDER.

This recipe makes a dentifrice which is similar to the all white tooth powder sold in boxes or bottles, and frequently in bulk by the quantity.

This formula makes an all white powder which is equal to any of them; there is actually no better than that made by following recipe:

Take

   Pure Precipitated Chalk, } each 4 ounces.
     "   Pulv. Drop Chalk, }
     "   White Sugar, 3 ounces.
     "   Cuttle Bone, 1 "
     "   White Castile Soap, 2½ ounces.
     "   Borax ½ ounce.
  Oil Wintergreen, 2 drachms.
    ' Sassafras, ½ drachm.

Mix the powders together; then add the oils gradually, and rub them together until they are thoroughly commingled.

This powder may be used every day or as often as it is required to keep the teeth all right.

CAMPHORATED TOOTH POWDER.

This recipe makes a tooth powder which is perhaps less used than some of the other kinds.

This of course does not make it an inferior powder; it is largely due to its not being so wellknown as some of the other preparations, and to the fact that some people object to the odor of camphor. It is, however, a very efficacious dentifrice, and is often preferred to any other.

It certainly will keep the teeth in good condition and give the mouth a very fresh, healthy taste.

Take
Pure Precipitated Chalk, 4 ounces.
Pulv. White Castile Soap, 1 ounce.
"   Camphor Gum, ½ ounce.
"   White Sugar, 1 ounce.

The camphor used here must be very finely pulverized; then mix the powders all together until they are thoroughly commingled.

Directions for using.—Apply it just the same as any of the other tooth powders.

PREPARATIONS FOR THE TEETH IN LIQUID FORM.

The market is overflowing with a great many different preparations for the teeth in liquid form under all manner of names which are being lauded as new discoveries for which wonderful claims are made.

Of course this should be taken with a little allowance, there will be no difficulty whatever for anybody who has this book to make a preparation in the liquid form,

or any other, which will in every way be equal and
probably superior to any of them.

This class of dentifrices are designed to be used as
a wash for the teeth, gums and mouth, and may, therefore, be used quite freely and frequently, or at least
once every day; they will help to preserve the teeth
by removing all injurious substances from them; and
restore or keep the gums in a healthy state by the healing and soothing properties they possess. Above all
they are very pleasant to use. They will give to the
mouth and breath an agreeable and lasting odor. A
little used upon a soft brush on the teeth and gums
after meals will leave a very pleasant, sweet taste in
the mouth; and remove any substance that may have
lodged between or on the teeth. This is indispensable
after eating; otherwise such substances will become
foul, and undergo decomposition, by which the teeth
will suffer and become affected, causing decay and final
loss of them.

THE ARCADIAN DENTIFRICE.

A VERY SUPERIOR PREPARATION IN LIQUID FORM.

I desire to call particular attention to this recipe; it
is a preparation for the teeth that I have put up a great
many times for friends who have always pronounced it
one of the very finest they ever used. I positively
know that it is an effective and delighfully pleasant
preparation to use.

I would suggest to those that have been in the habit
of buying some of the expensive preparations, to give
this one a trial. I feel confident that if they do so, they
will be convinced that it is unsurpassed. Above all,

they will have a full knowledge of its constituents,
which is a matter of considerable satisfaction to everybody who uses any of the various preparations for the
teeth. To make the ARCADIAN—
Take

Ground Soap Bark, ½ ounce.
Red Castile Soap, 2 drachms.
Pulv. Borax, 2 drachms.
Pulv. Cochineal, 10 grains.
Alcohol, 4 ounces.
Pure Glycerine, 4 ounces.
Pure Water, 8 "
Oil Cinnamon true, ⎫
    " Anise seed, ⎬ each 6 drops.
    " Wintergreen, ⎭
    " Sassafras, ⎫
    " Cloves, ⎬ each 6 drops.
    " Peppermint, ⎭

Cut the Castile soap in small pieces, and put all the
ingredients in a bottle for eight days; shake it
thoroughly once or twice each day; at the end of the
eight days strain it through a fine cloth, or pour it off
without disturbing the sediment.

The appearance of the Arcadian can be improved
greatly by filtering it through paper instead of straining or pouring off. Filtering paper can be had at any
drug-store.

Directions for using :—Saturate the tooth brush with
pure water; then pour on a small quantity of the
Arcadian Dentifrice, and brush the teeth thoroughly
until they are well cleaned. If one application proves
insufficient, repeat the operation until the desired result is obtained; then rinse the mouth with pure
water.

THE "IOKAH."

FOR THE TEETH.

This recipe also makes a beautiful preparation for the teeth; it will improve, preserve and beautify them, and give to the mouth and breath a delightful aroma, and a fresh healthy feeling which is very much appreciated. It seems to tone up the gums and leave the mouth in a healthy state.

Take
Pure White Castile Soap, ½ ounce.
" Glycerine, 2 ounces.
Pulv. Borax, 2 drachms.
Alcohol, 6 ounces.
Pure Water, 8 ounces.
Tincture Cochineal, plain, 1 drachm.
Oil Anise Seed, ⎫
" Sassafras, ⎬ each 10 drops.
" Spearmint, 2 "
" Sweet Orange, 15 "
" Wintergreen, 10 "

Shave off the white Castile soap in small pieces; then dissolve it in the water; mix the borax with the glycerine; shake together well; then add it to the solution of soap. If necessary, a little heat may be used in dissolving the soap. Add the oils to the alcohol; then mix all together and shake very hard for a short time; when this has been done, add the tincture cochineal, and shake all together thoroughly; then allow it to stand still for two days. If there should then be any sediment, pour off the clear liquid or filter through paper; then keep it well corked.

Directions for using the " *Iokah* ":—Put a few drops

on a tooth-brush which has been previously well moistened with pure water, and brush the teeth well; after they have been cleaned thoroughly, rinse the mouth with pure water. If this is used lightly every day it will give tone, vigor and strength to the teeth and gums. I feel confident that it will give the very best satisfaction.

THE WHITE ROSE DENTIFRICE

IN LIQUID FORM.

This preparation is entirely different from the ordinary run of these liquid compounds. It has features not possessed by others, though it is not a universal favorite. It has a beautiful rose flavor, to which many persons are somewhat partial.

Take
Pure Glycerine, 2 ounces.
"   White Castile Soap, 3 drachms.
"   Carbonate Potassa, 8 grains.
"   Water, 4½ ounces.
"   Alcohol, 2½ "
Extract White Rose, 1 drachm.
"   Cochineal, 40 drops.

Cut soap up in small pieces; dissolve it in the water; then add the alcohol and carbonate potassa; shake well together; then add the extracts Rose and Cochineal; shake again vigorously, and allow to stand still for two days; then if there is sediment in the bottom of the bottle either pour off the clear liquid or filter through paper, in order to have a fine, bright, clear looking preparation when finished.

Directions.—Apply to the teeth by putting a small quantity on the brush, which must be previously moistened with pure water. This may be repeated several times if necessary, to thoroughly clean the teeth.

Any of the foregoing liquid preparations for the teeth may be used upon artificial teeth with the most gratifying results.

Artificial teeth require attention as well as the natural teeth do. Therefore do not neglect them; all who have them should be very particular about keeping the teeth and plate clean. The plate especially should be carefully looked after. There is no way this can be done more effectively, than by the use of one of the liquid dentifrices for the teeth which can be made from the recipes in this book. It is a positive fact that they will make superior, or just as good preparations in every way as those that are sold in the market at such exorbitant profits as to make some of their proprietors enormously rich. In order to satisfy yourself on this question, I simply ask you to have some of the preparations made up properly and from best quality materials and compare them with any of the preparations of similar character you may have been using.

ANTISEPTIC LOTION.

This preparation is intended more especially as a mouth wash, for tender gums or sore mouth, although it may also be used for cleansing the teeth and gums. It will render the breath sweet, pleasant and fragrant, and keep the teeth, gums and mouth in a healthy condition.

Take

Tincture Myrrh, 3 drachms.
"   Kino, 1   "
Fluid Extract Orris-root, 1 ounce.
Pulv. Boracic Acid, 10 grains.
Pure Glycerine, ½ ounce.
Oil Peppermint,   ⎫
"   Sassafras,   ⎬ each 5 drops.
"   Cloves,   ⎭

Dissolve the boracic acid in the glycerine; add the tinctures and extract orris, then the oils, and shake all together thoroughly.

Directions for using.

Shake well, then add from 20 to 30 drops of the · lotion to a tumbler of pure water, then rub the teeth and gums with a brush saturated with this wash. Use only a soft tooth brush, wash the mouth thoroughly by rinsing a number of times with the wash or diluted lotion. The wash may be made stronger, if desirable, by adding 20 to 30 drops more of the lotion.

This wash imparts a pleasant odor and gives vigor to the gums. It must be left to the discretion of each person how often to use it. Ordinarily two or three times a week are sufficient in alternation with your regular dentifrice.

DENTIFRICES IN PASTE FORM.

Some people prefer a dentifrice in this form to any other. It has its advantages, and is a very nice preparation to use, when it is made from materials that are entirely free from deleterious substances.

AROMATIC TOOTH PASTE.

The preparation that is made after this recipe will answer all the requirements of a first-class paste dentifrice, and will be acceptable to those desiring a dentifrice in this form. It has all the good properties that the tooth preparations in liquid or powder form possess, and is used with equally as much gratification. It preserves the teeth, gives tone and vigor to the gums, and a very pleasant and lasting fragrance to the mouth and breath.

Take
Pulv. Orris Root,   2 ounces.
"   Drop Chalk,   4   "
"   Cuttle Bone, 1   "
"   Gum Myrrh,   ½   "
"   " Acacia,   ½   "
"   Red or White Castile Soap, 1 ounce.
"   Cochineal, 2 drachms.
Oil Cloves,
"   Peppermint,
"   Sassafras,
"   Wintergreen, each 10 drops.
Ess. Oil Bitter Almonds, 3 drops.
Pure Glycerine sufficient to form the whole into a
    stiff paste.

Mix the powders all together; add the oils, and again thoroughly mix them. Then add enough of the pure glycerine to form it into a very stiff paste. Put in a box or jar and keep it well covered.

Directions for using :—This should be used by taking a small quantity of the paste upon a dry tooth brush; then moisten the brush with pure water, and lightly brush the teeth and gums a number of times; lastly, rinse the mouth with pure water.

This paste keeps the teeth and gums in a healthy condition. Do not brush the teeth too hard nor use a very stiff brush.

COMPOUND CHARCOAL TOOTH PASTE.

This recipe makes a popular preparation. Some, however, do not like it, principally because the color is too dark for them. It will positively prevent and arrest decay in the teeth; improve the gums; and whiten the teeth without affecting the enamel. When its merits become known, it is much sought after for the apparently magical effects it produces upon the teeth. It will whiten and beautify them quicker than the majority of preparations which are used for this purpose.

Take
   Pulv. Willow Charcoal, 1 ounce.
      " Castile Soap, 2 drachms.
      " Cuttle Bone, 1 drachm.
      " Flor Orris root, 4 drachms.
   Oil Anise Seed, 5 drops.
    " Cloves, 3 drops.
    " Sassafras,
    " Sweet Orange, each 12 drops.
   Pure Strained Honey, ½ ounce.
    " Glycerine, about 1 ounce.

Mix the powders; add the oils, and rub well together, in order to get it well mixed; then stir in the honey. After this is done, stir in enough of the glycerine to form the mixture into a stiff paste; the amount of the glycerine required varies; it will be well to go slow, make the paste just right. Do not have it too dry; as it will dry out some itself. Put it into a well covered box or jar.

Directions for use :—Put as mall quantity of it upon a tooth brush, wet with pure water, then apply to the teeth andgums, and give them a gentle rubbing; this may be repeated at such times as may be necessary to keep them in proper condition. After they have been brushed, the mouth should be rinsed well with pure water. It will leave a very pleasant odor in the mouth.

PART III.

THE FINGER NAILS.

The finger nails should be very carefully and properly attended to.

This matter, I am pleased to note, is receiving the close and careful attention it deserves from the people, especially those who understand how much it improves the appearance of the whole hand to have the nails properly manicured. Everybody ought to adopt the means of having finely shaped and nicely polished finger nails. This may be easily done, as all the appliances can be purchased for successfully treating them, and it does not require much experience to enable those who have some tact to do justice to their hands. I have known a great many persons who after manipulating the fingers a few times have been agreeably surprised to see how well they performed the operation. After a little experience it becomes comparatively easy to manicure the fingers fully as well as it is done by most of the so-called professionals or experts in the art of manicuring. All that is really necessary is to procure at your drug or notion store, a good manicure set and use the following nail powder, in connection with brush, file, polisher, and other appliances which come with the manicure set.

This treatment will most assuredly produce gratifying results, if done carefully and thoroughly, so as to bring the condition of the fingers and nails up to their highest stage of perfection, giving beauty to the tapering fingers, polish to the nails, and natural perfection to the hand.

The market is full of different nail powders, from which great results are promised; but none of them are better than can be made from the following recipe when properly put up from good materials.

MANICURE POWDER.

Take

Pure Pulv. Drop Chalk, 1½ ounce.
" " French Chalk, 1 ounce.
" Cuttle Bone, ½ ounce.
" Pumice Stone, ½ drachm.
" White Castile Soap, 1½ drachm.
" Carmine, 5 grains.
Oil Sandal Wood, ½ drachm.
" Neroli Petale, 10 drops.
" Cloves, 5 drops.
" Bitter Almonds, 2 drops.
" Extract Musk, 20 drops.

7

Prepare this as follows :

The powdered ingredients must be the very finest pulverized ; rub well together, in order to thoroughly mix them; then add the oils and extracts which should be previously mixed together; stir gradually and continuously until it is all thoroughly mixed.

Keep this powder in a bottle or box tightly covered up.

Directions for using Nail Powder :—It may be used in the dry state, or it may be moistened before it is applied. Employ only a small brush which is made especially for this purpose. Take a little of the dry ' powder upon the brush and apply it to the nails, brushing them thoroughly ; then use the nail-polisher or a small piece of chamois skin; bear on hard and rub briskly; this will produce a beautiful polish.

When moist powder is to be used, moisten the brush in water, and put some of the powder upon it; then rub it over the nails several times, until they are nicely cleaned. Finish with the polisher as above.

This treatment should be followed up regularly ; and the change which will take place in the appearance of the whole hand when it is properly manicured will be very gratifying and will positively pay for the labor and time in doing it.

BATHING POWDER.

This powder will be of the utmost service to those who live where they have only hard water to use. I have often put up this recipe for people who wanted something which would render hard water soft and fit

and use only such quantity as may be necessary to
bathe in. It is an exceedingly fine preparation to
make water soft. Those having tender and delicate
skin are enabled to bathe in the hardest kind of water,
providing they put a small quantity of this powder into
it, without the least danger of their skin becoming all
rough and chapped, as it does when they attempt to
bathe in the hard water. The addition of this powder
at once renders the water soft, and also gives to it, and
consequently to the body, a delightful perfume, which
it retains for some time. Water treated with this powder is very cooling and healing to the skin, and leaves
a soft feeling on the surface. The face, neck, hands
and arms should be bathed in it freely, for it renders
the surface soft and smooth, and prevents chafing and
chapping.

Take

Pulv. Bicarbonate Soda, } each 4 ounces.
 " Borax,

 " Salts Tartar, } each 1 drachm.
 " Muriate Ammonia,

Oil Bergamot,
 " Cloves,
 " Sassafras,
 " Rose Geranium, } each 10 drops.
 " Wintergreen,
 " Lavender,
 " Anise Seed,

Mix the powders together thoroughly; then mix the
oils together also. Then gradually add the oils to the
powder, and keep stirring until it is all incorporated.

The Salts of Tartar should be pulverized before
being added to any of the other powders; otherwise

you will not get a fine powder. This combination should be kept in a bottle with a wide mouth, tightly corked.

Directions for using.—Add a very small quantity to the water, and allow it to dissolve before using it. When desired for use in bath water, put a small quantity into the bath-tub; then allow the water to run in, and stir if necessary, to dissolve it.

Soap should be used just the same as though the water had not been treated with this preparation. A less quantity will, however, produce in this water a much better suds. Use only a good quality of soap. Dry the skin thoroughly when the bath is completed.

PART IV.

HAIR PREPARATIONS.

A well-preserved head of hair on a person of middle age at once bespeaks refinement, elegance, health and beauty. But how often do we meet with people who have lost nearly all their hair long before that age has been reached! Why is it so?

I positively assert that ninety per cent. of it is caused by inattention and neglect. This matter deserves the serious consideration of everybody—those who have so far been able to retain all the natural beauty of the hair, as well as these unfortunates who have lost about all they had, and others who have perhaps neglected their hair until it has become dry and harsh, and is turning prematurely gray and falling out, while the scalp is full of dandruff.

All this may be overcome, the hair preserved, improved and beautified, and the scalp be thoroughly freed from dandruff, by using some of the following preparations for the hair and scalp. The variety of recipes to select from will give all an opportunity to find just what they need for the hair and scalp.

COMPOUND QUININE TONIC

FOR THE HAIR.

The following formula will make a preparation that I have put up more or less for a long time: I have found that in some cases when the hair seemed bound to fall out, that this proved to be one of the best preventives ever used. There is nothing better for giving strength and vigor to the hair and tone and vitality to its weakened roots. If the life is not entirely gone from the roots it will produce a heatlhy growth of hair on any bald head in a short time. It will also keep the scalp free from dandruff. In some obstinate cases it must be used faithfully for a long period. Do not get discouraged, for the result is tolerably sure if the roots of the hair are not dead; when they are, it is beyond mortal power to produce a growth, notwithstanding the statements to the contrary by some of the wise people.

To make the Compound Quinine Tonic—

Take.

Bisulphate Quinine, 40 grains.
Pure Glycerine, ½ ounce.
Best Bay Rum, "   "
Spirits Lavender Comp, 3 drachms.
Tincture Red Saunders, 1½   "
    "   Cantharides,   4   "
Pure Water, 5 ounces.
Cologne Spirits, 8 ounces.
Extract Jockey Club, 2 drachms.
Oil Bergamont,
    " Cloves,
    " Rose Geranium,   } each 6 drops.
    " Wintergreen,
    " Sassafras, 3 drops.

Prepare as follows :

Mix the cologne, spirits and water together; then dissolve the quinine in it by shaking hard; then add all the oils. Mix the bay rum, glycerine, tinctures and extract together; then combine the two mixtures and shake thoroughly. Filtering will improve its appearance very much, though it is not actually necessary.

Directions for using.—Apply to the scalp; be sure to get it down to the roots of the hair. In bad cases it should be used every day; in others every second day or once or twice a week.

The scalp should always be well brushed with a dry hair brush before putting it on ; then rub on well with the palm of the hand or flat part of the fingers ; never use the finger nails. The rubbing should be kept up long enough to considerably excite the scalp, in order to get up a brisk circulation.

When desired, this preparation may also be used as a hair dressing.   Apply a small quantity lightly each day.

HAIR VITALIZER.

This preparation imparts a rich gloss to the hair and renders it fine and soft. It also gives health and tone to the capillary glands ; prevents the hair from falling out; stop premature grayness, and gives strength to weak hair.

Take

    Pure Jamaica Rum, 6 ounces.
    Pure Grape Brandy, 2   "
    Tinct. Peruvian Bk. plain, 2 ounces.
    Alcohol, 5 ounces.
    Pure Cryst. Castor Oil, 1 ounce.
    Acetic Acid, 2 drachms.
    Oil Alspice, 10 drops.
    " Bergamont,   } each ½ drachm.
    " Lavender Flow. }
    " Lemon, fresh, 1 drachm.

Dissolve the oils in the alcohol; add the acetic acid, grape brandy, Jamaica rum, and tincture bark.

Directions for using.—Shake well before using ; apply it to the hair and scalp every other day as long as required ; rub it on hard with palm of the hand.   It can also be used as a hair dressing, and works very nicely on the beard or mustache.   Try it; the effects are pleasing.

THE HAIR TONIC AND PRESERVER.

I have put up this recipe a great many times. It imparts vigor to the roots of the hair; thoroughly cleanses the scalp, and eradicates all dandruff; it stops the hair falling out and, through its stimulating properties there is a healthy action of the scalp produced by which the whole condition is changed; thus securing continued growth of the hair and preventing baldness.

Take

Tincture Blood Root, } each ½ ounce.
    "   Cantharides, }

Pure Glycerine, } each 1 ounce.
    "   Crystal Castor Oil, }

Pulv. Carbonate Ammonia, 1 drachm.
Alcohol, 12 ounces.
Bay Rum, 4   "·
Extract Heliotrope, 2 drachms.
Oil Bitter Almonds, 5 drops.
    " Rose Geranium, 1 drachm.

Add the oils to the alcohol; dissolve the ammonia in the bay rum; then add the glycerine to it; then unite the two mixtures and shake well together.

Directions for using. — Always shake the mixture well before using; apply it to the hair and scalp quite freely and rub it on hard for some time with the palm of the hand to get it down to the roots of the hair. It may be used every day or every third day, according to the case.

"FLOUNCING FLUID"

FOR CURLING THE HAIR.

This recipe makes a preparation that is very much

admired, and it is just the thing for people who desire to have curly hair.

Take

> White Gum Arabic, 1 drachm.
> Pulv. Borax. 2 drachms.
> Spirits Camphor, 1 drachm.
> Best Cologne, 4 drachms.
> Alcohol, 3 drachms.
> Pure Water, 7 ounces.

Dissolve the gum arabic and borax in the water; then add the cologne, mix the camphor spirit with the alcohol, and add the two mixtures together.

Directions for using.—Just before retiring at night moisten the hair with the fluid and roll into twists with paper, leads or other devices, in the usual manner. After they have been rolled up long enough, generally over one night, take down and curl.

This fluid may also be used for making frizzes, bangs and the numerous other styles of curls.

COCOANUT OIL HAIR DRESSING.

This recipe makes a preparation which stands high with the people, for it is truly an elegant dressing for the hair; it renders it soft, beautiful and vigorous, preserves its luxuriance, supplies the roots with the properties which are very essential to their life and without which the hair ceases to grow and gradually falls out.

Take

> Pure Fresh Cocoanut Oil, 1 ounce.
> " Alcohol, 8 ounces.

Best Bay Rum, 6 ounces.
German Cologne, 1 ounce.
Pure Glycerine, 1 ounce.
Oil Neroli Petale, 10 drops.
" Sandal Wood, 15 drops.
Pulv. Carbonate Ammonia, ½ drachm.

Add all the oils to the alcohol and shake well together; then add the bay rum—in which the ammonia should be dissolved—and shake up thoroughly; then add the remainder. Perhaps the cocoanut oil will settle to the bottom of the bottle, more or less; that however will not change or affect its medicinal properties. When it is to be used simply give it a good shaking and it will all commingle. It separates mostly when the temperature gets down.

Directions.—This dressing may be used as often as required to keep the hair and scalp in a good, healthy condition. Do not put on too much at one time; a little of it goes a good ways; always rub on hard and spread over the surface thoroughly.

AN ELEGANT HAIR DRESSING.

This formula makes a perfect dressing for the hair; it promotes its growth, preserves and beautifies it and renders it soft and glossy. Few preparations possess the peculiar properties which so exactly suit the various conditions of the human hair. When the hair is impoverished this supplies nourishment on which it seems to thrive and become once more strong, healthy and beautiful.

Take
Pure Castor Oil, 2 ounces.

Tincture Blood Root,
    "   Cantharides, each ½ ounce.
Best Bay'Rum, 1 ounce.
Oil Lavender Flowers, ½ drachm.
  " Rose Geranium, 20 drops.
  " Sweet Orange, 1 drachm.
  " Lemon, fresh, 15 drops.
Extract Jockey Club, 2 drachms.
Alcohol, 12 ounces.

Dissolve the oils in the alcohol; add the bay rum and the tinctures; then the extract jockey club.

Directions.—Apply to the hair and scalp; rub it on hard with the flat part of the fingers or with the palm of the hand. It may be applied every day, or as the condition of the hair suggests. Do not put on too much at one time; a medium quantity applied often and well rubbed in serves better. It is suitable for old or young.

POMADE CREAM FOR THE HAIR.

This recipe makes a combination that will, when properly used, in many cases entirely cure baldness. It is also an excellent dressing for the beard or mustache. It softens the hair, gives it lustre and soothes the irritated scalp. Its effects are permanent.

This preparation can be carried when you are traveling, without danger of soiling the clothing.

Take
Rose Cosmoline, 4 ounces.
Bals. Peru, 1½ drachms.
Sulphate Quinine, 25 grains.
Oil Cade, ½ drachm.
  " Rose Geranium, ½ drachm.
  " Bitter Almonds, 5 drops.

Mix the quinine with the balsam of Peru; then add this to the rose cosmoline, with all the other ingredients; mix them all together.

Directions for using.—Take a small quantity on the fingers or into the palm of the hand, and put it upon the hair or scalp, rubbing sufficiently to oil it well. Do not use too much at one time, as it might be too oily. Apply each day or every two or three days. For the beard or mustache apply with the fingers a small quantity only, and spread it out well. It has a beautiful effect upon the beard.

"GLYCEROTINE"

FOR DRESSING AND BEAUTIFYING THE HAIR AND BEARD.

This recipe also makes an elegant dressing for the hair, producing the most remarkable effects. It renders it very beautiful and gives to it a rich lustrous appearance.

This effect cannot be secured from any of the ordinary hair dressings.

Take

    Pure Glycerine, 2 ounces.
    White Rose Cologne, 2 ounces.
    Tincture Kino, 15 drops.
    Oil Sandal Wood, 10 drops.
    Alcohol, 2 ounces.
    New England Rum, 2 ounces.

Add the tincture kino to the glycerine; then the white rose cologne; mix the oil sandal wood with the alcohol and New England rum; then unite the two mixtures, and shake well.

Direotions for using.—Whenever a beautiful lustrous appearance is desired for the hair, this is the preparation to use. Put on a little of it only at a time, and spread it out well over the hair. Use it as often as you need it.

BRILLIANTINES.

This class of preparations are used principally for enhancing the beauty of the hair. An occasional application of the *Brilliantine* will keep the hair soft, silky and bright looking, dispelling that dead appearance which it sometimes presents. In order to give it a brilliant, rich, lustrous appearance, use the Brilliantine; it will not disappoint you.

The following recipes I have used considerably. Do not hesitate to employ them, as the results will certainly be gratifying.

AMERICAN BRILLIANTINE

FOR BEAUTIFYING THE HAIR.

Take
   Best pure Olive Oil *fresh*, 3 ounces.
   Pure Alcohol, 1 ounce.
   Oil Neroli Petale, 20 drops.
   " Bitter Almonds, 2 drops.
   " Bergamot, ½ drachm.
   Otta Rose, 4 drops.
Mix all together.

This preparation will separate after standing a while.

Directions for using. —Always shake thoroughly before applying it. Put on lightly, and spread it well over the hair. It acts charmingly on the beard or mustache. Just a little applied to the hair every day or two will keep it looking fine.

"FRENCH BRILLIANTINE"

FOR DRESSING AND BEAUTIFYING THE HAIR, BEARD OR MUSTACHE.

How often do we hear people say this or that preparation which they use for toilet purposes is **French**, and is therefore superior to anything and everything else? The time, when that was true has passed by; for now with the right formulas and first quality of materials, we can make just as good right at home as can be made abroad.

The matter of greatest importance is to have a reliable recipe, then have it properly put up from the freshest and purest materials. When this is done and the instructions carefully followed, the product will be equal to any, wherever made. I claim that this is the case with the various recipes in this book; they will make first class preparations when properly put up from only the best materials.

The result will be a combination equal to any, and superior to a great many.

For French Brilliantine take

Pure Olive Oil fresh, 1 ounce.
" Alcohol, 3 ounces.
Oil Rose Geranium, 10 drops.
" Lavender Flowers, 10 drops.
" Bay Leaves, 10 drops.
" Cinnamon Tree, 5 drops.
" Sandal Wood, 15 drops.

Mix the oils together, then add the alcohol.

Directions for using.—This preparation must always be well shaken when applied; spread it thoroughly but lightly over the hair occasionally; it will give it a beautiful, silky, lustrous appearance. Gentlemen will find this an elegant dressing for the beard or mustache. It will improve their appearance wonderfully.

THE MABEL BRILLIANTINE

FOR IMPROVING AND BEAUTIFYING THE HAIR.

This recipe makes an exceptionally fine preparation. It is very highly esteemed by those who are acquainted with its qualities. It certainly has no superior for giving to the hair a beautiful appearance. There is nothing disagreeable about it; on contrary, it is a very delightful preparation to use.

Take

Pure Glycerine, 2 ounces.
Pulv. Borax, 1 drachm.
Cologne Spirits, 4 ounces.
Best Bay Rum, 1½ ounce.
Best Extract Musk, 2 drachms.
Oil Ylang Ylang, 20 drops.

Dissolve the borax in the glycerine; add the spirits (in which the oil has been dissolved); then add the other ingredients, and shake all together.

Directions.—Shake well before using. Spread it on evenly. It keeps the hair in splendid condition. Do not put on too much at one time.

It will be noticed that the Brilliantines are different in composition. Some people will like one and some another kind. My object in giving so many different preparations is to satisfy all and enable each person to gratify their taste in this matter. I have learned from experience that it is actually necessary to do this, and I trust there will be enough to go around. All are good preparations, and can be made by anybody with the knowledge obtainable from this book.

In making any of the Brilliantines, use only the best, freshest and purest goods. A poor quality of material will impair the effects of the preparations and do injustice to my recipes, and to those using them.

SEA FOAM.

FOR CLEANSING THE SCALP AND HAIR FROM ALL IMPURITIES.

This preparation is somewhat similar to shampoos; but it has its own peculiar properties and merits. The results obtained through its use are very beneficial.

Take

    Pure Alcohol, 8 ounces.
    Pure Water, 7 ounces.
    Aqua Ammonia, ½ ounce.
    Carbonate Ammonia, 1 drachm.
    Tincture Gentian Comp., ½ ounce.
    Best Cologne, 1 ounce.

Dissolve the carbonate ammonia in the water; add the alcohol and other ingredients.

Directions for Using.—This preparation should be used perhaps once a week or once in two weeks, according to the condition of the hair and scalp. Use it just enough to keep the hair and scalp in a cleanly condition.

Apply the sea foam to the scalp in quantity sufficient

to produce a copious lather. Pour a small quantity at a time right on the head, or into the palm of the hand first; then rub the head and hair hard and brisk with the flat part of the fingers and the palm of the hand.

If this treatment fails to produce a copious lather, put a little water on the head. It is necessary for the person using it to exercise some judgment as to the strength of the lather required to produce the best results. After it is in good working order the rubbing of the scalp may be continued until the lather all disappears; then thoroughly dry the head and hair with a dry towel.

When it is used by the ladies they must have their hair thoroughly dried before doing it up. Always use soft water. If the hair should become too dry and crispy use one of the hair dressings made from my recipes.

This preparation will prove very beneficial to either ladies or gentlemen, and keep the hair and scalp in excellent condition.

SHAMPOOS.

Shampoos are all used in about the same way. They differ more or less in composition; but the rules for using one applies to all of them, and can be substantially followed with satisfactory results. Apply all to hair and scalp thoroughly; wetting them, and rubbing hard and brisk enough to produce a thick, heavy lather. When it is found that the shampoo smarts sharply and irritates the scalp, it will be a good plan to reduce it with water, either before using or on the head.

Reducing it on the head is considered the best; (always use soft water). Pour the shampoo on the head; if it fails to work, pour on water, rubbing steadily until it works up a good stiff lather. If the shampoo prove too weak, it can be made stronger by adding ammonia.

The shampoos made after the formulas in this book are as good as any; they are perfectly harmless, and will positively be a benefit to the head, scalp and hair. I advise people who are troubled with headache to try a shampoo often. I have seen some excellent results from its use; it will frequently give immediate relief.

There are a great many different kinds of shampoos in the market; but after many trials I found the preparations here given proved as satisfactory as any combinations that are put together. Some contain a large amount of soap, which causes the preparation to thicken up, and it is then used in the form of a cream. There is, however, no advantage in this; when it is wanted, there is nothing better to use than the pure White Castile Soap; wash the head and hair thoroughly with it, then rinse out well, dry it, and apply some hair dressing.

SHAMPOO EUREK__

FOR THE HAIR AND SCALP.

This preparation is especially adapted to the use of the ladies. What gives more relief or is more appreciated by the ladies, than to have the head thoroughly shampooed, especially during hot weather. To have the hair and scalp thoroughly freed from dandruff, and the dust that settles upon it, must indeed be a favor as well as a pleasure. In this book I have given all the recipes for making the various preparations which are so necessary to comfort and happiness, without obliging the ladies to go to the hair-dresser, which is frequently so disagreeable a task that it is put off for a long time, until the hair suffers serious injury.

Select the dressing you may desire to use, procure the materials and prepare it yourself, or have it prepared at the drug store. This makes it easy for anybody to take a shampoo at home. To make the Eureka shampoo,—

Take
    Cologne Spirits, 6 ounces.
    Tinct. Blood Root, 2 drachms.
    Salts of Tartar, 2 drachms.
    Aqua. Ammonia, 1½ ounce.
    Extract Frangipani, 2 drachms.
    Extract Jockey Club, 2 drachms.
    Water, ½ pint.

Mix the water and alcohol together; then dissolve the salts of tartar in it; add the other ingredients, and keep it well corked.

Directions for using.—The shampoo should be used at least once a week in summer time; during the winter season perhaps once in two weeks will be sufficient to keep the hair and scalp thoroughly cleansed.

Apply it first to the scalp. Wet it thoroughly in soft water; then rub hard with flat of fingers or palm of the hand, until it soaps up nicely. Continue this treatment until the scalp is well cleansed; then, apply the shampoo to all the hair in similar way. Then thoroughly rinse off with clean water, and dry the head with a towel. If it becomes too dry and fluffy after being shampooed, use one of the hair dressings lightly the day after using the shampoo.

If the above shampoo fails to produce a good soap-suds, add some water to it on the head, as in using the Sea Foam; or if it is too strong and sharp reduce with water. This will no doubt produce the right effect.

SHAMPOO FOR GENTLEMEN.

This preparation is especially adapted to the use of gentlemen. It requires no special training to use it. You can do it yourself as well as an experienced barber.

If this shampoo is used once or twice a week during summer time, it will keep the scalp and hair in excellent condition and the head cool. All have realized the advantage and comfort of this.

There is just one drawback which prevents a great many availing themselves of this soul-stirring and brain soothing treatment: that is going to the tonsorial artist to have the operation performed. This too often proves so tiresome and perplexing that a great many forego the benefits to be derived rather than to submit to the annoyance. With the aid of this book any gentleman may have all the benefits without the annoyance. It will enable him to procure the proper materials to make his own shampoo, and give him the necessary instructions how to prepare and use it. Then there will be no temptation to deprive himself of the luxury. Besides, he may have the satisfaction of enjoying its benefits as often as he desires.

The following recipe makes a shampoo that I have

put up for barbers as well as for private use during a number of years, and it has always given the very best satisfaction.

In my experience behind the Drug-Store counter, I have found that, whenever I made a preparation which failed to please the person buying it, it did not take long for him to let me know it. · Hence I soon learned whether an article was approved. The recipes in this book, I have put up, more or less, for nearly twenty years ; the verdict generally has been a smile of satisfaction on the countenance of the parties using them. This gave me the key to the situation at once, and enabled me to talk with confidence about the preparations, because I had this sure way of proving their excellence. I am confident gentlemen using this shampoo will say that it is as good, if not better than any other ever used.

Take
    Pure Water, 6 ounces.
    " Alcohol, 7 ounces.
    Carbonate Potassa, 2 drachms.
    Aqua Ammonia, 1½ ounce.
    Pure Glycerine, 1 ounce.
    German Cologne, 1 ounce.
    Extract Jockey Club, 2 drachms.
    Tinct Benzoin, plain, 20 drops. ·

Mix the alcohol and water, dissolve the carbonate potassa in it ; then add the glycerine, cologne, ammonia, extract and benzoin ; shake well together and keep tightly corked.

Directions for using.

Shake well and apply to the head ; give it a thorough rubbing, until it produces a heavy lather. If this fails to form after a quantity has been put on the head and well rubbed in, put some water right on the head with the shampoo preparation, and rub all together. After the head has been rubbed hard, and the hair and scalp thoroughly cleansed, rinse it off with pure water; then thoroughly dry the head, and apply a little good strong bay rum. Next day, if necessary, use a little hair dressing.

The shampoo may be used as often as necessary. When the above course is followed, the hair and scalp will be kept free from dandruff, itching and other disturbing features. In reducing shampoo use soft water.

BRILLIANT HAIR DRESSING.

This preparation will materially improve and beautify the hair. It has a splendid effect after using the shampoo or sea foam; for it will soften the hair when dry or harsh from lack of natural oil, and give it a permanent lustre.

Take

  Pure Glycerine, 1 ounce.
  New England Rum, 2 ounces.
  Rose-water, 4 ounces.
  Dist. Ext. Witch Hazel, ½ ounce.
  Extract Jockey Club, 2 drachms.
      "   Frangipani, 2 drachms.

Mix all the ingredients together.

Directions for using.

This preparation may be applied as often as necessary, to keep the hair in the condition desired. Put on only just enough to spread over the hair; too much of it would spoil the effect. It has a splendid effect upon the beard or mustache, making it glossy and silky, when used not oftener perhaps than once in two or three days.

PERUVIAN HAIR TONIC.

This recipe makes an extraordinary dressing to assist the growth of the hair and beautify its appearance. If used occasionally it will prevent its falling out, and have a refreshing effect upon the scalp.

Take
 Balsam Peru, 4 drops.
 Pure Castor Oil, 4 drachms.
 Tinct Jam. Ginger, 2 drachms.
 " Camphor, 2 drachms.
 New England Rum, 4 ounces.
 Pure Alcohol, 4 ounces.
 Oil Bitter Almonds, 5 drops.
 " Bergamot, ½ drachm.
 " Lemon, ½ drachm.
 " Cloves, 3 drops.

Add the oils, balsam Peru, spirits, camphor and tincture ginger to the alcohol; then add the New England rum and shake all together.

Directions for using.

Brush the scalp thoroughly with a good stiff hair brush; then shake the tonic well and apply to the scalp and hair lightly every day or two; rub it on hard with palm of the hand.

DANDRUFF ERADICATOR.

This recipe makes a preparation which will positively remove all dandruff and scurf from the scalp, and also prevent its formation. Its effects are highly appreciated by those who are acquainted with its merits.

Take

Pulv. Carbonate Ammonia, } each 2 drachms.
    " Borax, }
Sulphate Zinc, 5 grains.
Peppermint-water, 4 ounces.
Glycerine, 1 ounce.
Brandy, *Pure*, 1 ounce.
Alcohol, 2 ounces.
Pure Water, 8 ounces.
Oil Bay Leaves, 10 drops.
    " Cloves, 5 drops.
Rose Geranium, 10 drops.

Dissolve the borax, zinc and ammonia in the plain water; add the peppermint-water; dissolve the oils in the alcohol; add the brandy and glycerine; then put the two mixtures together, and shake up well.

Directions for using.

Apply the eradicator to the scalp every day until there is no more dandruff or scurf on the head. It should be well rubbed on with the flat part of the fingers and the palm of the hand.

If the case is of long standing, and the scalp has become very sore, do not rub hard enough to produce irritation, but apply the eradicator gently for a short time. Persevere in its use—no matter how long the difficulty has been going on—and you will be rewarded by a lasting cure.

If on the start the eradicator smarts considerably, reduce it with water; after it has been used a short time the smarting will be overcome.

"BANDOLIN."

Very few ladies are unfamiliar with the word Bandolin.

The following recipes will make Bandolin in every way equal to the higher priced article.

The ladies will find the Bandolin made after the recipes following to work perfectly as an aid in dressing the hair in the various fashionable styles.

BANDOLIN POWDER.

For making liquid Bandolin take
  Pulverized Gum Tragacanth, 2 ounces.
  " Borax, ½ drachm.
  " Soap Bark, 20 grains.
  Oil Rose Geranium, ½ drachm.
  Otta Rose, 3 drops.
  Oil Cinnamon Tree, 4 drops.
  " Bitter Almonds, 2 "
  Extract Musk Tincture, ½ drachm.

The preparation in liquid form is the one always used on the hair.

A very fine liquid preparation may be made from the Bandolin powder. Have the powder on hand, and when Bandolin is wanted it can be made on short notice.

LIQUID BANDOLIN.

Can be made from this powder by adding two teaspoonfuls of the powder to half-pint of water. Warm water will hasten the completion. Agitate it occasionally until all the powder is taken up, then press it through cloth, in order to give it a better appearance. If it is too thick add more water; if too thin more powder.

Directions.

Mix the powders together; then add the oils and extract, which should be previously mixed gradually. Keep stirring until thoroughly commingled. Put into a bottle which must be dry. Keep in dry place, well corked.

BANDOLIN

IN LIQUID FORM.

This recipe will make a very fine preparation for staying the hair; it is positively equal to any of the expensive imported ones. It has an elegant odor, which is very delicious and lasting. It is no trouble to make it nor does it require any knowledge beyond that which is given in this work, which is simplified to such an extent that it only requires some tact and a little time to produce a Bandolin the effects of which will actually surprise you.

Take

 Best quality Quince Seed, 6 drachms.
 Pure Glycerine, 1 ounce.
 Plain Water, 7 "
 Alcohol, 1   "
 Extract Jockey Club, 2 drachms.
  " Wood Violet, 2 "
 Oil Sandal Wood, 10 drops.

Add the quince seed to the water; let them stand together 24 hours; then strain through muslin; add the glycerine and extracts; dissolve the oil in the alcohol, and add that; then shake all together.

In using Bandolin preparation the time and quantity must be left discretionary; put on only such an amount

as is actually necessary. If too large a quantity is used
it will be apt to show in a white substance on the hair.

HAIR RESTORERS.

The following recipe makes a preparation similar to
those usually sold as *Hair Restorers,* for which such
wonderful claims are set forth. Those who believe
the advertisements actually imagine that something
new has been discovered instead of the same old thing
with slight variations served up under a new guise. I
do not sanction the use of this character of preparations, for they all are more or less injurious and deleterious in the end.

A great many people, however, think differently,
and insist on using them. Therefore as the public will
have them, I have concluded to place a formula here,
which will make a Hair Restorer that can be used with
as little danger as any of the so-called Hair Restorers;
besides this has the advantage of showing just what is
the nature of the composition. But I repeat that I do
not sanction the use of any preparation of this character.

Take
  Sugar of Lead, ½ ounce.
  Lac Sulphur, 6 drachms.
  Table Salt, 2 drachms.
  Jamaica Rum, 4 ounces.
  Aqua Ammonia, 2 drachms.
  Alcohol, 2 ounces.
  Pure Glycerine, 1 ounce.
    " Rain Water, 1½ pints.

Extract Jockey Club, 2 drachms.
    "   Frangipani, 2   "
Oil Bergamot, 5 drops.
  " Rose Geranium, 5 drops.

Mix the sulphur, lead, ammonia and alcohol together, and let them stand 12 hours; then add the other ingredients to the water and mix all together; then shake it thoroughly and let it stand **four days** before using it.

Directions for Using.

After the mixture stands several hours there will be a heavy sediment at the bottom; this should not be disturbed, but apply to the hair the clear liquor from above the sediment. Thoroughly moisten the hair with the liquor, and allow it to dry, the hair meantime being left loose. Repeat this process as often as you think prudent, to keep the hair in its natural color. From one to six times a week is ordinarily enough in the start; afterwards an occasional use will prevent the hair turning gray.

In applying this restorative it is quite important to wet the hair thoroughly, in order to produce the desired result.

PART V.

HAIR DYES.

This is also a class of preparations I never could sanction, as I am satisfied that they are also detrimental to health. It is therefore only to meet a positive demand that I give the following recipes, which I have frequently put up for people who insisted on using them. I will give only the most harmless of any that can be used for this purpose.

I learned long ago that life is too short to show everybody the folly of his ways, so I contented myself with serving out the most harmless combinations for the above purpose that skill and experience could put together.

The following is a recipe for making a hair dye:

NUMBER ONE DYE.

Take
    Pyrogallic Acid, 30 grains.
    Pure Water, 1½ ounce.
    " Alcohol, ½ "
Mix the alcohol and water together; then dissolve the acid in it. Keep in bottle well corked.

NUMBER TWO DYE.

Take
    Pure Nitrate Silver, 1½ drachms.
    " Water, 6 drachms.
    Aquæ Ammonia, 2 drachms.

Prepare by dissolving the silver in the water—*distilled water is the best*—first—never dissolve the ammonia first, as that would spoil the dye. When it is dissolved, add the ammonia, which should be strong enough to re-dissolve the precipitated silver. If the materials are strictly pure and as strong as they should be, the result will be a perfectly clear solution, which will however become dark, on standing. This will not affect the properties of the dye. If the ammonia used is weak, a larger quantity will be required to re-dissolve the blackish looking precipitate which forms, and to leave an entirely clear liquid.

Directions for Using the Hair Dyes.

Ladies must thoroughly cleanse their hair by using either aqua ammonia and water mixed in the proportion of about one ounce ammonia in a pint of water ; or some shampoo which does not contain any oil or glycerine. Then carefully rinse it, to get out all the soap and lather. To have the dye take good, it is necessary that it should be completely freed from all oily or greasy matter. After it is washed it must be well rinsed with clear water, and allowed to dry. The hair will then be ready to use the dye upon it. When both the No. 1 and No. 2 preparations are used, follow these instructions :

First apply the No. 1 solution with a small brush or sponge to the hair only ; none should go on the scalp. It can be done very nicely, by holding the hair upon a comb away from the scalp; this will prevent any of the solution getting on the skin. After all the hair has been treated with the No. 1 solution allow it to dry. Then apply the No. 2 dye with a small tooth brush, and a comb to hold out the hair as above directed.

The dye must be applied to the hair very carefully ; do not allow any to get upon the scalp or skin. When the preparations are both carefully put on and thoroughly dried, the hair becomes perceptibly darker.

After the dye has set, wash the hair with pure soap and water ; afterwards it should be well dried, and some nice dressing lightly applied to it.

When the dye preparations are made from good quality of material and put on according to these instructions, you will notice, just as soon as the No. 2 preparation comes in contact with the hair that has the

No. 1 solution on, that the effect is immediate; the change takes place at once, producing a jet black color.

In applying the solutions, do not put on very much at a time; just a small quantity each time until the hair has all been touched with them. If any gets on the skin, it is very difficult to remove the stain, but the following will generally do it : Get a piece of Sulphuret Potassa at a drug-store, and moisten it with a little water; then apply it to the stain, or spot. It may be necessary to repeat the operation several times.

After the stains have been removed, wash off with plenty of water; do not use any soap with the Potassa. Caution in putting on the dye will prevent its getting on the skin.

The hair, beard or mustache, whichever has been dyed, should be washed out thoroughly with soap and water; this should not be neglected.

I have always found that if the parties using these preparations were very particular to get the hair free from all oily and greasy substances, the first application would be satisfactory. But if the dye don't take after several applications, the fault is to be ascribed to poor materials, or bad preparation and treatment.

Gentlemen using the dye for the hair, mustache or beard must use it in the same way. First, thoroughly wash the hair to be dyed ; then, apply the No. 1 preparation with a small brush; allow it to dry; then apply the No. 2 preparation in the same way with a separate brush. If the shade produced is not dark enough, the dye may be applied the second or even the third time in the same way.

The hair dye must be used often enough to color the hairs as they grow out; the growth varies so much with different people that no more precise instructions on this point can be given.

HAIR DYE WITH ONLY ONE PREPARATION.

I have put up this preparation a great many times for people who preferred to use one dye. I always found that this recipe would give splendid results when properly handled. It will produce a shade of brown, by simply adding a larger amount of ammonia, the shade varying with the amount of the ammonia that the dye contains. When black is desired, the ammonia must be reduced; when a brown shade is preferred, the amount of ammonia must be increased.

This single preparation can be used with equally satisfactory results by both Ladies and Gentlemen.

Take

Pure Nitrate Silver, 1½ drachm.
Pure Water *distilled*, (if it can be had) 4 drachms.
Aqua Ammonia, 4 drachms.

Dissolve the silver in the water *first;* this must always be done, or the dye will prove a failure. After it is dissolved add the ammonia, which must make a clear solution; otherwise, more or stronger ammonia must be used to clear the mixture.

After adding the ammonia a change takes place that will throw down the silver in the form of a blackish brown sediment, and this must be re-dissolved with the ammonia. This can be done very readily.

The ammonia should not be too strong, or else the effect of the dye would be impaired. It must be only just strong enough to re-dissolve the precipitate which forms.

Directions for using.

Follow the instructions given under the preceding hair dye recipes in every detail, up to where the hair is ready for the dye. The latter is the all important thing in connection with the quality of the dye, which in turn hinges upon the materials being only the very best.

This preparation should be applied to the hair with a tooth brush; hold the hair up on a comb to prevent staining the skin. Let it dry after each application, and apply a sufficient number of times to produce the desired shade. Remove stains on the skin as directed on previous page.

If the hair is exposed to the rays of the sun after the dye has been applied the latter will take hold much faster than if allowed to dry in the ordinary way.

PART VI.

BAY RUM.

This delightfully refreshing preparation is used more or less by people throughout the civilized world, and is very highly prized for its medicinal properties as well as for the pleasant aroma it possesses. When applied to the surface it produces a most agreeable, cool sensation. There is perhaps no one thing that holds the

9

place among toilet requisites that bay rum does. There is always much variation in quality; a great deal which is sold is hardly worthy of the name.

It is certainly a matter of considerable importance to the consumer to know that the bay rum is of good quality; but a high price does not always assure a good article.   This can be secured beyond doubt by buying your own materials from reliable parties.   The following recipe will make a bay rum that is in every respect equal to the genuine imported bay rum, and far superior to a great deal that is sold as such.

I have sold bay rum made from this recipe for a number of years, and always found that it gave satisfaction.   Of course it is not a distilled bay rum, but it has a very much pleasanter aroma and is more lasting.

Bay Rum equal to the Imported.

Take
 Best Oil Bay Leaves, 1 drachm.
  " " Allspice, ⅔ drachm.
  " " Nutmegs, 10 drops.
  " " Cloves, 15 drops.
  " " Sandalwood, 20 drops.
 Acetic Ether, ½ ounce.
 Pure Glycerine, 1 ounce.
 Extract Vanilla, true, 2 drachms.
 Pure Jamaica Rum, 4 ounces.
  " Water, 5 ounces.
 Acetic Acid, 1 drachm.
 Pure Alcohol, 21 ounces.

Dissolve the oils in the alcohol; add the acetic acid and ether; shake well, then add the Jamaica rum, glycerine, vanilla and water; now shake it all together thoroughly and let it stand three days.   If cloudy, filtering will make a beautiful clear liquid; or, if not convenient to filter, the clear liquid can be poured off from the sediment. It could be used just as it is, but the filtering improves its appearance very much, though not its quality. Only the best and freshest material should be used in making these bay rums.

The above recipe really makes an elegant bay rum.

It is without question considerably stronger than the majority of bay rums that are sold. If too strong, weaken it with water.

BAY RUM (GOOD QUALITY).

This recipe will also make a very satisfactory combination. It is of good strength, lasting, and very agreeable. It compares favorably with other preparations.

Take
Pure Oil Bay Leaves, 1 drachm.
" " Allspice, ½ drachm.
" " Cloves, 10 drops.
Extract Musk, true, 1 drachm.
Acetic Acid, 1 drachm.
Jamaica Rum, 2 ounces.
Pure Alcohol, 23 ounces.
" Water, 6 ounces.

Dissolve the oils in the alcohol; add the rum, extract musk, acetic acid and water; shake all well together; let it stand four days; then filter if necessary; keep it corked up tight to preserve the aroma.

BAY RUM (WITH AMMONIA).

This makes a bay rum which differs from the general run; it has peculiar properties which others do not possess; the addition of a little ammonia increases its pungency. Some prefer it to any other kind, on account of its being extra strong. When a very refreshing, pungent and agreeable bay rum is wanted, I would suggest this, made after the following recipe:

Take
> Pure Oil Bay Leaves, 1 drachm.
> " " Bergamot, 20 drops.
> " " Pimento, ½ drachm.
> New England Rum, 2 ounces.
> Glycerine, 1 ounce.
> Aqua Ammonia, 1 ounce.
> Alcohol, 24 ounces.
> Water, 4 ounces.

Dissolve the oils in the alcohol; add the New England rum, glycerine, ammonia and water; shake well together and let it stand four days; it may then be filtered if desired.

If you want a bay rum, or in fact anything for which recipes are furnished, select the one you want prepared, take it to a druggist and have it put up; or get the materials called for and prepare it yourself. It will be equal to any of the high-priced preparations if my instructions are followed.

BAY RUM

FOR GENTLEMEN.

This recipe makes a bay rum truly superb, to use after shampooing or shaving. There is something that seems peculiar to this particular combination. In some instances it may be a little too strong, and smart on the face too much to be comfortable. When such is the case reduce it with water to suit.

Most gentlemen like a bay rum that will take hold sharp; they generally find it a difficult matter to get any such at the barber shops. To be independent of the barber's bay rum (at 5 cents extra), select the particular recipe that you may like, and make a bay rum that costs less, but is worth more money.

The particular bay rum made after this formula will prove very satisfactory, as it is much pleasanter to use than the ordinary kinds. It also gives to the heated skin during the summer season a very cooling and refreshed feeling. It would be difficult to find its superior.

Take
    Pure Oil Bay Leaves, 1½ drachm.
    "   " Pimento, ½ drachm.
    "   " Sassafras, 10 drops.
    Ottar Roses, 2 drops.
    Acetic Ether, ½ ounce.
    Spirits Lavender Comp., ½ ounce.
    Pure Glycerine, 1½ ounce.
    Pure Water, 4½ ounces.
    Alcohol, 1 pint and 9 ounces.

Dissolve the oils in the alcohol; then add spirits lavender comp., acetic ether, glycerine and water; shake together thoroughly, then let stand three days. It may be filtered, but this is not actually necessary; it adds to the appearance, but not to the quality of the rum.

BAY RUM, (ORDINARY).

The following recipe will make a very fair quality for general use ; it is considerably cheaper than any of the others for which recipes are furnished ; but it makes a very desirable rum and is just the thing for common every-day use, where the question of expense comes into consideration.

Take
    Pure Oil Bay Leaves, 1 drachm.
      "   " Allspice, 1 drachm.
      "   " Cloves, 20 drops.
      "   " Bergamot, 15 drops.
    Glycerine, 1 ounce.
    Acetic Acid, 2 drachms.
    Jamaica Rum, 4 ounces.
    Alcohol, 2½ pints.
    Water, 1½ pint.

Dissolve the oils in the alcohol ; then add the glycerine, acetic acid, Jamaica rum, and lastly the water ; shake all together thoroughly and let stand four days. If filtering through paper fails to bring it out nice and clear, it should be filtered through powdered carbonate of magnesia ; place this right in the bottle containing the bay rum ; then proceed to filter just as though there was no magnesia in, except that it must be well shaken before it is poured upon the filter ; if it does not come out clear the first time it passes through the filter, run it through again. This may be repeated as many times as necessary to bring the rum through bright and clear. It will take from 1 to 2 ounces of magnesia for the whole amount of the recipe.

It will be noticed that all the recipes for making bay rum have a similarity ; yet each one has peculiarities of its own. Of course, the particular ingredient to which all bay rum owes its prominent odor is the oil contained in, and procured from, the leaves of the bay tree, and generally called oil of bay. The other ingredients are added to vary the character of it, and also to suit conditions of demand ; they all affect the result.

The formulas in this book are the results of my experimenting with different combinations ; they have all been used and thoroughly tried for a number of years, and the popular verdict is that they possess all the good qualities I claim for them. They will positively prove satisfactory, and you will at the same time be saving money.

_____

PART VII.

TOILET WATERS.

This is a subject every refined lady and gentlemen is deeply interested in.

The following recipes produce toilet waters which are much superior to a great many of those that are sold.

They will produce perfumed water which will at once suggest to a person a bouquet of flowers in bloom ; their odor can only be equaled by that of the natural flowers. What is more delicious or can start the imagination quicker, than the fragrant odor of one of these beautiful toilet waters !

It will, so to speak, take a person right in among a thousand different beautiful flowers, where their exquisite odor may be inhaled.

I respectfully submit my recipes for making the different toilet waters to an exacting public, feeling satisfied the universal verdict will be that they are not excelled by any.

Any of these perfumed or toilet waters may be used in the sick room, where they often exercise a beneficial influence upon the invalid. There is something so hopeful and refreshing in them that the patient is inspired with confidence in the future.

The paper which comes made for filters can be obtained from the Druggist, who will show you just how to fold the filter, for use.

The filter paper comes cut in circular form; it is generally folded once, making a half circle. Fold it over and over until it is made into folds about an inch wide at the top; then open it out and place it in a funnel; it will readily shape itself to the sides of the funnel. Be careful not to break the point of the paper while folding it. Place the funnel in the bottle and pour the liquid into the filter slowly; if put in suddenly and in large quantity the filter would be very apt to break. Keep adding more until all the liquid has been passed through the paper filter. Sometimes it is necessary to do this more than once. When it is properly done, the result is a beautiful, bright, clear, sparkling preparation.

This rule applies to all liquid preparations which require filtering.

In preparing these toilet waters use only the best materials; otherwise the completed preparation will disappoint you.

HELIOTROPE WATER.

FOR THE TOILET.

This recipe makes a very fine preparation, and gives general satisfaction.

Take
    Ess. Oil Bitter Almonds, ½ drachm.
       " Rhodium, 20 drops.
       " Rose, pure, 5   "
       " Rose Geranium, 1 drachm.
       " Neroli Petale, ½ drachm.
    Extract Vanilla, true, 1 ounce.
    Fluid Ext. Orris Root, 1 ounce.
    Extract Musk, true, 3 drachms.
    Extract Civet, 1 drachm.
    Rose Water, 1 ounce.
    Pure Alcohol, 1 pint.

Prepare by dissolving all the oils in the alcohol; then add the extracts and lastly the water. Shake well together and let it stand three days. If it becomes cloudy run it through a filter paper to clear it up.

This toilet water may be used in about the same way that cologne waters are used.

The above is a very superior preparation; a small quantity added to the bath water will produce a delightful effect, and give to the skin a fragrant odor.

VIOLET TOILET WATER.

The market is full of preparations by this name; some are very fine, but extremely high-priced, or else of poor quality.

The following recipe produces a violet water which will stand comparison with the very best, while the majority cannot begin to equal it for fragrance and lasting qualities. Therefore, when a violet water is desired which possesses all the most desirable features, do not hesitate to use this one.

Take

     Oil Ylang Ylang, 10 drops.
     " Cinnamon, true, 20 drops.
     " Lemon grass, 20 drops.
     " Cloves, 10 drops.
     " Bergamot, 1 drachm.
     " Lavender Flowers, $\frac{1}{2}$ drachm.
   Extract Violets, $\frac{1}{2}$ ounce.
   Fluid Extract Orris Root, 1 ounce.
   Benzoic Acid, $\frac{1}{2}$ drachm.
   Rose Water, 1 ounce.
   Peppermint leaves, 1 drachm.
   Alcohol, 14 ounces.

Prepare by dissolving the benzoic acid and all the oils in the alcohol; then add the extracts, rose water, and peppermint leaves, shake well together and let it stand four days, during which time it should be shaken twice a day; then filter through paper as above, or pour off.

FLORIDA WATER.

This Toilet requisite is so well known it is sufficient to say that this recipe will make a Florida Water equal to any.

Take

     Oil Sweet Orange, 2 drachms.
     " Bergamot, 2 drachms.

Oil Lavender Flowers, 2 drachms.
" Neroli Petale, 2 drops.
" Rose Geranium, 20 drops.
" Cinnamon, true, 10 drops.
" Cloves, 10 drops.
" Sandal Wood, 15 drops.
" Pimento, 5 drops.
" Lemon grass, 5 drops.
Chloroform, 1 drachm.
Rose Water, 1 ounce.
Cologne Spirits, 14 ounces.

Prepare as follows :

Dissolve the oils in the cologne spirits, add the chloroform and rose water, shake well and let stand four days, when, if necessary, filter ; this of course only is done when the preparation has stood the four days and has become cloudy; when filtered it will clear it up and improve its appearance.

FRENCH LAVENDER WATER.

This recipe will make a Lavender Water that will in every way be equal to the imported French preparation ; it is exceedingly fragrant, lasting, and very refined; it has been a great favorite with people who have used it. It is made as follows :

Take

Oil Lavender Flowers, 4 drachms.
" Bergamot, 1 drachm.
" Lemon, fresh, 1 drachm.
" Cloves, 5 drops.
" Rose, pure, 3 drops.
" Civet, 20 drops.
Extract Ambergris, ½ drachm.

Balsam Peru, 1 drachm.
French Spirits, 15 ounces.
Orange-flower Water, 1 ounce.

Prepare as follows :

Mix the oils, balsam Peru, and extract ambergris with the French spirits, and shake well ; then add the orange flower water and repeat the shaking; then let it stand four days. If it becomes cloudy, filter it as above directed. If necessary some.powdered carbonate or calcined magnesia may be added to it in the bottle before filtering. This is very strong, but not rank, as it is beautifully blended.

AMERICAN LAVENDER WATER.

This recipe makes a favorite preparation. It is very agreeable and lasting, and produces a genteel and delicate odor. It can be had by having the following combination put together:

Take

Oil Patchouly, ½ drachm.
" Lavender Flowers, ½ ounce.
" Cloves, 15 drops.
" Winter-green, 15 drops.
" Bay Leaves, ½ drachms.
" Ylang Ylang, 10 drops.
Benzoic Acid, 1 drachm.
Orange Flower Water, 1 ounce.
Best Alcohol, 1 pint.

Prepare by dissolving the benzoic acid and the oils in the alcohol ; then add the orange flower water ; shake together well and let stand five days ; then it may be filtered.

This is a very pleasant perfume to add to the bath water; it makes the greatest improvement imaginable in the effect the bath has upon the skin.

"THE AMBER" LAVENDER WATER.

This recipe makes a preparation which has considerable color. Many people hold it in high esteem, and use it in preference to any perfumery.

When a very fine amber water is desired this can always be relied upon. It is equal to any of the expensive preparations of this character on the market. The materials must, of course, be the very best and freshest. There actually are few toilet waters which are used with more genuine gratification than this one. When bathing add a small quantity to the water in which the bath is to be taken. This is where its good qualities are brought out to the best advantage.

Take
Oil Sandal Wood, 1 drachm.
" Lavender Flowers, 4 drachms.
" Rose Geranium, 1 drachm.
" Sassafras, ½ drachm.
" Cassia, 20 drops.
" Cloves, 20 drops.
" Nutmegs,
" Allspice, each, 15 drops.
" Patchouly, 20 drops.
Extract Vanilla, true, 2 drachms.
Tincture Red Saunders, 4 drachms.
Extract Musk, true, 4 drachms.
Rose Water, 1 ounce.
Cologne Spirits, 1 pint.

Prepare as follows :

Dissolve the oils in the spirits; add the extract, tincture red saunders, and lastly the rose water; then shake well and let it alone four days; then filter, if necessary, to have it come out bright and clear. Use it whenever Amber Lavender Water is desired.

———

" VERBENA TOILET WATER."

This recipe makes a combination that commands the admiration of those who use it. It has lasting properties that are very striking, and is also very pleasant and a little different from the majority of this class of preparations.

Take

    Pure Fresh Oil Verbena, 1½ drachm.
    Glycerine, 1 ounce.
    Oil Lemon Grass, 8 drachms.
    " Lemon, fresh, 1 drachm.
    " Neroli, ½ drachm.
    Fluid Extract Orris-root, 1 ounce.
    Extract Tonka Beans, ½ ounce.
    Rose Water, 1 ounce.
    French Spirits, 1 pint.

Prepare as follows :

Dissolve the oils in the spirit; then add extracts and rose water; shake well together; then let it stand four days; then, if it requires it, filter through paper.

Keep well corked. Use as desired, same as cologne or perfumery.

" THE FRANKLIN TOILET WATER."

This recipe makes a toilet water the name of which is no doubt new to most readers.

It is one I have put up for some time; it has always met with the highest praise and was very much appreciated.

I therefore submit the recipe with the feeling that it will find a place among the most popular preparations. The combination is as follows:

Take
Oil Ylang Ylang, 20 drops.
" Cloves, 16 drops.
" Thyme, pure, 10 drops.
" Bitter Almonds, 5 drops.
" Verbena, pure, ½ drachm.
" Rose Geranium, 1½ drachms.
" Lavender Flowers, 2½ drachms.
" Canada Snake Root, ½ drachm.
" Nutmegs, fresh, ½ drachm.
Extract Musk, 2 drachms.
Tincture Tolu, 3 drachms.
Chloroform, ½ drachm.
Rose Water, 1 ounce.
Cologne Spirits, 1 pint.

Prepare as follows:

Dissolve all the oils in the spirit; then add the chloroform, tincture tolu, extract musk and rose water; shake well together; then allow it to stand quiet for six days; after which filter it sufficient to bring it out bright and clear.

This perfume will be found a most exquisite and delightful toilet water.

TOILET OR AROMATIC VINEGAR.

This is a preparation highly prized by people who are acquainted with its merits. It has a very cooling and soothing effect when applied to the skin. It is often used as an application to the head, and will allay headache, and that feeling of faintness which is at times so troublesome to control.

It may also be used in the sick chamber with the most beneficial results. Applied to the forehead, it will refresh the patient, and induce much needed rest for the almost worn out sufferer, who will wake up with new hope and courage.

Toilet or Aromatic Vinegar has been used a great many years, and many people are well acquainted with its medicinal properties, as well as its great merits as a toilet preparation, to those who are not familiar with it, I would recommend the following recipe for Aromatic Vinegar:

Take
Pulv. gum Camphor, 1 drachm.
Oil Lemon fresh, 1 drachm.
" Lavender flowers, ½ drachm.
" Cloves, 25 drops.
" Lemon-grass, 4 drops.
Tincture, Benzoin plain, 1 drachm.
"   Storax, 1 drachm.
Extract Tonka true, 1 drachm.
Fluid Extract Orris Root, 1 drachm.
Acetic Acid, 1½ ounce.
Rose Water, 2½ ounces.
Cologne Spirits, 12 ounces.

Prepare by dissolving the oils and camphor gum in the spirit; then add the tinct. benzoin, storax, and tonka; shake together; then add the other ingredients, the rose water last. Finally give it all a good shaking; let it stand quiet four days, when it may be filtered.

Directions for using.

Apply it to the surface of parts affected; it may be used as a liniment by rubbing it on lightly, or a cloth can be saturated with it and laid on to the affected place.

When it is wanted for inhalation a small sponge may be saturated with the vinegar, put into a smelling bottle, and used as vinaigrette. The latter mode is employed largely by people who suffer with frequent headaches or fainting spells.

The effect it has upon these maladies will surprise those who have never used it. It should also be applied to the forehead in conjunction with the inhalation for headache.

It can also be used to good advantage to odorize a room. The best way perhaps is to use an Atomizer, which with its fine spray, will odorize a room quicker and more perfectly than any other mode. Another way is to fill a dish with the vinegar and let it stand in the room; or saturate some cloths and suspend them in the room in different places. It can be done in any manner that will be the most convenient.

TOILET REQUISITES.

The selection of Perfumes, Toilet Water, Cologne, Bay Rum, Powders, Balms, Creams, Lotions, Hair Preparations, or any of the various preparations used in completing the toilet, must to a large extent be left to each individual's tastes and peculiarities. Therefore it would be unwise to undertake to lay down any rule to govern the matter.

I can frankly say, however; that this work will be of more aid in selecting the kind each person may want than anything else which has ever been offered to the public. It is composed of tried formulas originated by a thoroughly practical pharmacist of nearly twenty years' experience; these have been compiled with great care and are varied enough to enable all to find just what is wanted, together with an exceedingly large amount of practical and reliable information, suggestions, instructions and other matter of interest.

PART VIII.

COLOGNES.

This is a subject which a great many will be pleased to read a little about. If there is a class of preparations in which the public is more deceived I have yet to learn what they are. There is a vast difference in the quality of colognes; from the good grades which usually sell at exorbitant prices to the poor grade that never ought to be called cologne. Many of them are nothing but a weak mixture of about 15 per cent of alcohol and water, and a small quantity of cheap oils.

From the recipes following can be produced colognes

which will bear comparison with the best, whether domestic or imported.

This superior line of Colognes I have put up more or
less for a number of years. I have from time to time
improved upon them until in their present shape they
are gems by themselves. From the great variety here
submitted there should be no difficulty in finding a
Cologne which will possess the desired qualities, and
merit the approval of the most fastidious.

In making these Colognes the purest and freshest
material is absolutely necessary to insure good results.
An impure or old essential oil will completely upset the
best formula that was ever written.

When these recipes are prepared from good material
they produce first class preparations that will be satisfactory in every particular.

BEGY'S FAVORITE COLOGNE.

I trust my readers will not consider me extra vain in
giving my name to the following recipe for making this
cologne.

I think I am justified in doing so, for this particular
recipe is one for which I have on several occasions
refused to accept a considerable sum of money. As
long as I remained in the drug business, I refused to
sell my recipes after giving up the business I concluded to publish this book, on which I had been working for a long time and decided to put only my very
best formulas in it. This cologne recipe is one of them.

Begy's favorite cologne can always be relied upon as
an elegant, delicate, yet lasting application.

Take.

 Oil Sandal Wood, yellow, 2 drachms.
 " Sweet Orange, 2 drachms.
 " Rose Geranium, ½ drachm.
 " Patchouly, 20 drops.
 " Bitter Almonds, 5 drops.
 " Ylang Ylang, 10 "
 " Rose pure,   3 "
 " Cloves,   10 "
 " Peppermint,   3 "
 " Anise Seed,   10 "
 Balsam Peru, 1 drachm.
 Butyric Ether, ½ drachm.
 Glycerine, ½ ounce.
 Rose Water, 1 ounce.
 Cologne Spirit, 1 pint.

 Prepare as follows :

Dissolve all the oils and balsam Peru in the spirit;
then add the butyric ether, glycerine and rose water;
shake all together; let stand quietly 4 days, then
filter and use as wanted.

NOTE.—After the colognes have been made and
allowed to stand the required time they will throw
down a precipitate to the bottom. This does not impair the cologne a particle, except in appearance; it
is objectionable, of course, to those who have been in
the habit of using cologne waters which are perfectly
clear. The remedy is to filter the colognes in the
same manner, substantially, as the Bay Rums. This
will give a finished cologne, as fine appearing as any
can be. I have always made it a practice to allow my
colognes to stand several days after they were made

before I filtered them; frequently when they are filtered as soon as the ingredients are put together they will throw down more or less sediment afterwards.

When a cologne is made up and allowed to stand for some time, before filtering, the finished cologne proves to be more satisfactory, and is more presentable, which I always found to be of considerable advantage in selling it.

Some of these colognes are made up from recipes which require no filtering, and can be used just as they are, or after being poured off. When filtering is necessary, and you are not inclined to do it yourself, it can be done by having the druggist put the materials together and filter it after letting it stand a few days.

ITALIAN COLOGNE.

This recipe makes a fine and lasting cologne. It is very sweet and fragrant, and will compare favorably with the high priced imported colognes. It will stand on its merits, and when once used, will be highly appreciated.

Take
Oil Neroli Petale, ½ drachm.
 " Lavender Flower, 2 drachms.
 " Bergamot, 2 drachms.
 " Cedrat, (citron) 1 drachm.
 " Sweet Orange, 1 drachm.
 " Sandal Wood, 1 drachm.
 " Cassia.
 " Cardamon Seed.
 " Cloves, each 10 drops.

Tinct. Tolu, ½ ounce.
True Grain Musk, 3 grains.
Butyric Ether, ½ drachm.
Water, 1 ounce.
Cologne Spirit, 1 pint.

Dissolve the oils in the spirit; add the tincture tolu, musk, ether and water; shake all together; then allow it to stand one week before filtering through paper; or if necessary to clear it, filter through the magnesia as directed in making bay rum.

SWEET ORANGE COLOGNE.

As the name implies, this recipe will produce a cologne that reminds one of oranges and orange groves so that it will be comparatively easy to imagine oneself in Florida among oranges and flowers. It is delicious to use; its sweetness is very much admired by people who desire a soft sweet cologne. It has none of the hard, harsh or coarse characteristics so common in a large number of colognes to which people of sensitive natures find so much objection.

Take
Oil Sweet Orange, 4 drachms.
" Neroli Petali.
" Lemon Fresh, each ½ drachm.
" Lavender Flower, ½ drachm.
" Anise Seed, ½ drachm.
" Bitter Almond, 5 drops.
" Cloves, 20 drops.
" Cinnamon, true, 5 drops.
Rose Water, 1 ounce.
Chloroform, ½ drachm.
Cologne Spirit. 1 pint.

Dissolve the oils in the spirit; add the chloroform, and rose water; shake well together, then let it stand four days; filter if necessary.

The above is a very fine perfume for indoor use, as it is fragrant and sweet.

NOTE.—It will be noticed that in a number of recipes for making colognes, bay rum and a few other preparations, the formulas call for cologne spirit. The very best alcohol, which is nearly free from fusel-oil and all impurities, is generally designated by this name, implying an alcohol purer than that commonly sold.

THE ORIENT COLOGNE.

The following recipe makes a cologne that is very strong and not quite as fine and delicate as some of the others. It is agreeable and pleasant, and no doubt it will find a great many admirers who will prefer it to any other.

This recipe will make about one quart. It will keep any length of time, but if this quantity is too large, reduce the ingredients to suit.

Take
    Oil Wintergreen, ½ drachm.
    " Lemon Grass, ½ drachm.
    " Bergamot, 3 drachms.
    " Lavender Flowers, 4 drachms.
    " Cloves, 1 drachm.
    " Cassia,
    " Sassafras, each ½ drachm.
    " Bitter Almonds, 20 drops.
    " Rose Mary, 1 drachm.
    " Rose Geranium, 1 drachm.

Oil Bay Leaves, ½ drachm.
Pulv. Camphor Gum 5 grains.
Pure Water, 5 ounces.
Alcohol, 28 ounces.

Prepare by dissolving the oils in the alcohol; then add the camphor and water ; then shake it all together and let it stand four days, after which it may be filtered. Keep in bottles tightly corked, and use as wanted.

AMERICAN COLOGNE.

This recipe produces a cologne that will cause the blood to tingle in the veins of all patriotic citizens who delight in home made products, and would no doubt delight the eagle if he could only have the opportunity of using it. Its beautiful flowery odor has no equal. It has all the essential elements of a first-class cologne.
Take

Oil Bergamot, 3 drachms.
" Rose Mary, ½ drachm.
" Red Cedar, 1 drachm.
" Lemon fresh, 1 drachm.
" Rose Geranium, 1 drachm.
" Orange Flowers, ½ drachm.
" Sandal Wood, 1 drachm.
" Wild Ginger Root, ½ drachm.
Benzoic Acid, 1 drachm.
Extract Musk, true, 2 drachms.
Rose Water, 1 ounce.
Cologne Spirit, 1 pint.

Prepare by dissolving the oils and benzoic acid in the cologne spirits ; then add the musk and rose water ; shake well tgether and let it stand six days, after which filter it.

GERMAN COLOGNE.

There are a great many colognes called German. Nearly all the druggists make it, besides selling numerous other kinds, both domestic and imported. The public is therefore familiar with this name as applied to colognes. There is a vast difference in them ; there are no two druggists who make it alike. Every one is peculiar to itself, and is generally as little like old fashioned German cologne as an artificial rose is like a natural one.

I tried a great many different combinations with varying success, until I finally produced the following, which from its very introduction seemed to be just what every lover of German cologne wanted. It possesses all the desirable features of this very popular cologne, without having any of the objectionable qualities so frequently met with in a large number of the so-called German colognes. I have no hesitation in saying that this is as good a German cologne as was ever made.

Take
    Oil Lemon-grass, ½ drachm.
    "   Sweet Orange, 4 drachms.
    "   Bergamot, 4   "
    "   Lavender flowers, 4 "
    "   Rose Mary, 20 drops.
    "   Neroli Petal, ½ drachm.
    "   Rose Geranium, 1   "
    "   Ceylon Cinnamon, 10 drops.
    Camphor Gum, 4 grains.
    Chloroform, ½ drachm.
    Extract Musk, 4 drachms.
    Butyric Ether, ½   "

Benzoic Acid, 1 ounce.
Rose Water, 1½ ounce.
Cologne Spirit 1½ pint.

Prepare by adding the oils, camphor, benzoic acid, and chloroform to the spirit shake well until dissolved, then add extract musk butyric ether, and rose water; shake quite briskly for a short time; then let it stand for six days, after which it may be filtered, if necessary.

PATCHOULY COLOGNE.

The following recipe makes a cologne in which the patchouly is the most prominent, a feature that is very much admired by lovers of this particular perfume. It has extraordinary lasting powers, for which a great many prefer it to almost any other kind. When, there-. fore, a patchouly perfume is wanted, one that will have lasting qualities without being rank, one that will be pleasant and fragrant, use this one.

Take
    Oil Patchouly, 1 drachm.
    " Rose Geranium, 1 drachm.
    " Cardamon Seeds, 20 drops.
    " Lavender Flower, 1 drachm.
    " Ylang Ylang, 10 drops.
    " Bergamot, 2 drachms.
    Extract Vanilla, true, ½ ounce.
    Orange Flower Water, 1 ounce.
    Cologne Spirit, 15 ounces.

This should be prepared by dissolving the oils in the spirit; then add the extract vanilla and orange water; shake up thoroughly; then let stand five days, after which if necessary filter it, and it is ready for use.

WHITE ROSE COLOGNE.

Among all the colognes there is none which can lay claim to being finer and more delicate than that made from the following recipe. It will positively make as fine a quality of 'white rose as any ever offered to the public. It has a sweet delicious fragrance that surprises a person when using it for the first time. Any one not familiar with such matters would hardly realize that such close resemblance to a bouquet of flowers in which roses predominate could result from this combination. But such is the case. There is not an atom of coarseness about it. It is a grand combination of refinement with good lasting qualities ; features which make it a favorite with both ladies and gentlemen.

In making it or having it made, use *only* the very best materials.

Take
  Pure Ottar of Roses, 10 drops.
  Oil Rose Geranium, 1 drachm.
  " Sandal wood, 1 "
  " Bay Leaves, 10 drops.
  " Ylang Ylang, 15 drops.
  Butyric Ether, ½ drachm.
  Extract of Musk, true, 2 drachms.
  Rose Water, 1 ounce.
  Cologne Spirits, 1 pint.

Prepare by dissolving the oils in the spirit ; it must be thoroughly shaken until all are dissolved ; then add the extract musk, butyric ether and rose water. Now give it another good shaking ; then keep it in a moderately warm place for four days, after which filter it; when it will be ready to delight all with its fragrant, flowery odor.

JOCKEY CLUB COLOGNE.

The following formula makes a cologne which is liked by nearly everybody. When you desire a good standard cologne, which is fragrant and refined in character, use the jockey club. The name jockey club as applied to perfumery is now quite old; the jockey club perfume has had an enormous sale, and is so well known that it is not necessary to enter into an elaborate description of its qualities. I trust the superiority of this cologne will be so manifest to those who use it, that the goods will talk for themselves.

This recipe makes a cologne that cannot be to highly praised. Give it a trial.

Take

Oil Lemon, fresh, 2 drachms.
" Lavender Flower, 2 drachms.
" Bergamot, 4 "
Oil Neroli Petale, 15 drops.
" Cinnamon, true, 5 drops.
" Cloves, 4 drops.
" Civet, 40 drops.
" Ambergris, 20 drops.
" Cedrat (citrons), 15 drops.
" Sweet flag, (calumus), 20 drops.
Otta Rose, pure, 3 drops.
Ess. Jasmin, 2 drachms.
Extract Musk, true, 2 drachms.
Orange Flower Water, 2 ounces.
Cologne Spirits, 29 ounces.

Prepare by dissolving the oils in the spirit; then add the extracts jasmine, musk, and the orange water, shake together thoroughly for a short time; then allow to stand 4 to 6 days; after this filter it, and use it to your heart's content.

THE MABEL COLOGNE.

The following recipe will produce a very superior cologne ; one that has some lovely features which cannot fail to be commended.

It has a most delicious fragrance. There are very few perfumes or colognes which surpass this one, when used in the bath, for it gives to the body a delightful odor not unlike perfumery. A small quantity put into the water in which the face, neck and hands are bathed, will produce a most remarkable effect upon the skin, making it very soft and velvety.

No lady will do without this exquisite toilet requisite after she has once used it, for it certainly is not excelled by any cologne in the world for softness and smoothness, especially when used in the water in which the bath is taken.

. Take
  Oil Sandal Wood, 3 drachms.
  " Lavender flowers, 3 drachms.
  " Bergamot, 4 drachms.
  " Bay Leaves, ½ drachm.
  " Ylang Ylang, 12 drops.
  " Cloves, 8 drops.
  " Sassafras, 16 drops.
  " Patchouly, ½ drachm.
  " Peppermint, 3 drops.
  Balsam Peru, 1 drachm.
  Pulv. Borax, 2 drachms.
  Glycerine, 2 ounces.
  Extract Musk, 2 drachms.
  Extract Vanilla, pure, 1 ounce.
  Chloroform, 1½ drachm.
  Rose Water, 2 ounces.

Cologne Spirits, 28 ounces.

Prepare this cologne by adding the oils, balsam, peru and chloroform to the spirit; then shake well together. Add the borax to the glycerine; dissolve by agitating it, and add the rose water after they have been shaken together. Combine the two mixtures; give all a brisk and thorough shaking up; then let it stand from four to eight days, when it may be filtered. If it does not clear up nicely of itself, put it through paper; then put about half an ounce pulv. charcoal right into the cologne; then pour on to the filter; and repeat until it comes out clear.

FRENCH COLOGNE.

The following recipe makes a cologne that closely resembles some of the most renowned French colognes. It is perfectly elegant; its fragrance is not surpassed by any. I can safely say this recipe will not lack admirers.

It has been repeatedly demonstrated that with a pure quality of materials we can make just as good colognes in this country as they do in France or elsewhere. The first element of success in doing so is to have a recipe that on trial will produce a first class grade of cologne.

The recipes in this book, come up to the above requirements; they are all of the same standard of excellence. Hence this book is worth its price many times over.

The French Cologne is made thus:

Take
  Oil Lemon fresh, 2 drachms.
  " Sweet Orange, 2 drachms.
  " Rosemary, fresh, 1 drachm.
  " Bergamot, 2 drachms.
  " Neroli Petale, ½ drachm.
  " Rose Geranium, ½ drachm.
  " Cloves, 10 drops.
  " Allspice, 20 drops.
  " Cardamon Seed, ½ drachm.
  True Grain Musk, 3 grains.
  Acetic Ether, 2 drachms.
  Cologne Spirits, 1 pint.
  Orange Flower Water, 1 ounce.

Prepare by dissolving the oils in the spirit; then add the musk, acetic ether and orange water. Shake all together thoroughly. Then allow it to stand for eight days, during which time it should be occasionally agitated; when the term has expired filter it through paper or if necessary through pulverized charcoal or magnesia, as previously suggested. When completed it will have a beautiful bright appearance.

PART IX.

SACHET POWDERS.

This particular feature will no doubt greatly interest the ladies, in this age of sachet powders, rose leaf jars, potpouri powder, and jars, and the other numerous artifices which are resorted to in order to perfume or odorize the house, the dressing case, trunk, bureau drawers, and other places which have to be taken care of. There are a large number of other purposes to which the sachet powders are well adapted, especially in the making up of fancy things in which a small amount of the powder adds to the attractiveness of the article.

The sachet powders sold in stores are quite expensive, but with the recipes for making them in your possession this will not be the case, and they can be used freely; without this advantage they are generally used sparingly on account of their expense.

NOTE.—In making the sachet powders it is only necessary to follow nearly the same instructions; what applies to one will be equally applicable to all of them. The subjoined recipes make sachet powders that will be well liked, and equal to any in the market, provided fresh material is used in making them. Any one of them may be used in the various jars, such as rose leaf, potpouri, and the various other kinds.

It is altogether a matter of preference as to which one is the best. They are all very strong and lasting; any one of them will no doubt give excellent satisfaction, for they all compare favorably with far more expensive preparations, either domestic or imported. When made from fresh material, there are very few powders that are equal to these. The general rule for making the different sachet powders is to follow these instructions:—When a recipe calls for an article to be ground, it should not be pulverized; but should be put in an iron mortar and pounded to the required fineness. This does away with the clogging of the mill in grinding the materials. It does not take long to pound, bruise and grind up the articles in the iron mortar. Do not grind too fine, and yet there should be no large pieces left in any article; it should all be about the same grade of fineness.

All the ingredients should be well mixed in order to get the most satisfactory preparations. This holds good in making sachet powders as well as in making the other preparations in this book. It is important to have everything just right before going ahead. All the ingredients should be fresh and of the best quality. Do not take anything else; insist on having them in this condition or not at all. Some of the ingredients called for may have been in stock a long time, and consequently have become almost inert. Never use these under any consideration, as it would prove detrimental and spoil the fine odor of the combination.

All sachet powders should be well sealed up when not in actual use; they will thereby retain their odor and strength a much longer period.

It will perhaps be a good plan when you want one of the sachet powders made up to have your druggist put it together for you, as he has all the necessary facilities for doing it; he can do it so much better than you, without much additional cost.

YLANG YLANG SACHET POWDER.

This recipe produces an elegant, very sweet and delicate powder, which is very much admired by people of refined taste.

Take
Ground Flor. Orris Root, 4 ounces.
" Gum Benzoine, ½ ounce.

Ottar Rose, pure, 5 drops.
Oil Ylang Ylang, ½ drachm.
" Sweet Orange, 1 drachm.
" Patchouly, ½ drachm.
Grain Musk, true, 5 grains.

Prepare by mixing the ground ingredients; then add the oils and musk, and thoroughly rub them together until the whole is thoroughly mixed.

DAMASK ROSE SACHET POWDER.

The subjoined formula produces a powder which has been used a great deal; it is a recipe from which I have made the powder for a number of years. It has always given the most decided satisfaction. I never hesitated to recommend it; I know the recipe will be liked, as the powder has all the elements necessary to make a good sachet.

Take

Ground Red Rose Leaves,   ⎫
    "   Yellow Sandal Wood, ⎬ Each 1 ounce.
    "   Flor. Orris Root,   ⎭
    "   Vanilla Bean, 2 drachms.
Oil Bergamot, 1 drachm.
    " Ylang Ylang, 15 drops.
    " Cinnamon, true, 5 drops.
Ottar Rose, pure. 8 drops.
Pulv. Camphor Gum, 2 grains.

Mix all the ground ingredients together; add the camphor; then rub them together well and add the oils gradually; keep stirring during the time the oils are being added. This should be very thoroughly mixed.

HELIOTROPE SACHET POWDER.

This recipe makes a heliotrope powder that is unsurpassed. I have sold as much, if not more, of this than of any other powder. It always has received very flattering praise from those using it.

Whenever you want a heliotrope powder, the odor of which resembles the flora, take this one. It will please you.

Take

 Ground Flor. Orris Root, 2 ounces.
  "   Red Rose Leaves, 4 drachms.
  "   Tonka Beans.
  "   Vanilla Beans, each 2 drachms.
 Best Grain Musk, 3 grains.
 Oil Civet, 10 drops.
 " Bitter Almonds, 5 drops.
 Otta Rose, pure, 3 drops.
 Oil Ceylon Cinnamon, 2 drops.

Prepare by mixing all the ground ingredients together; add the musk; then stir the whole up thoroughly; then mix the oils and gradually add them to the ground mixture; keep stirring the whole until they are well mixed. The more thoroughly this is done the better the sachet powders will be. The mixing divides the ingredients, and they become very evenly distributed. It is absolutely necessary to have the oils well distributed through the powder; this is really the secret of getting a sachet powder, with the perfume just alike all through it.

WHITE ROSE SACHET POWDER.

This powder is perhaps one of the most delicate among them all; yet as it is made from this recipe it is lasting. This is a very important matter with a white rose sachet; most of them do not hold their odor. I know from long experience with this recipe that the powder is very fine, delicate, lasting, and altogether a superb white rose.

Take
    Pulverized Flor. Orris Root, 3 ounces.
    Ottar of Roses, pure, 6 drops.
    Oil Rose Geranium, ½ drachm.
    "   Patchouly, 15 drops.
    "   Sweet Orange, ½ drachm.
    "   Ceylon Cinnamon, true, 2 drops.
    Grain Musk, true, 3 grains,

Prepare by adding the oils and musk to the pulverized orris root; then rub all together until they are completely commingled.

It will be noticed in these formulas for making the different sachet powders, that they nearly all contain orris root. It serves the purpose of a base and vehicle remarkably well, and being of a very agreeable odor it helps to make the combinations. Another consideration largely in favor of the orris root, is the fact that it is inexpensive.

The large profit to the manufacturer of some of the sachet powders consists in the cheapness of the orris root utilized in their composition. Some may think that on account of the orris being in all the different sachet powders, that they all resemble one another, and in odor and smell are too much alike. They will be agreeably surprised when I state that this is not the case. Every one of the recipes will make a powder which is peculiar to itself; they all have a character of their own.

PATCHOULY SACHET POWDER.

This sachet powder is a great favorite with some people. The recipe can always be depended upon for producing a combination that will have lasting qualities.

Take

    Ground Patchouly leaves, 1 ounce.

      "   Red Rose leaves, ½ ounce.

      "   Florentine Orris Root, 3 ounces.

    Pulv. Gum Benzoin, ½ ounce.

      "   Yellow Sandal Wood, ½ ounce.

    Oil Patchouly, 1 drachm.

      " Cloves, 15 drops.

      " Canada Snake Root, ½ drachm,

Mix all the ground ingredients; do the same with the oils; then add the oils to the ground mixture gradually; then add the powders and keep stirring and mixing until it is all thoroughly commingled.

BOUQUET SACHET POWDER.

This formula will produce a powder which is very fine and highly odorific. It is extra nice for odorizing rooms, by placing some of it in a powder jar.

Take

    Ground Yellow Sandal Wood, ½ ounce.

      "   Lavender Flowers, ½ ounce.

Ground Violet Flowers, ½ ounce.
"   Red Rose Leaves, ½ ounce.
"   Orris Root, 2 ounces.
Oil Ceylon Cinnamon, 20 drops.
"   Cloves, 15 drops.
"   Rose Geranium, ½ drachm.
Otta Rose, pure, 5 drops.
Oil Bergamot, 1 drachm.
"   Wintergreen, 20 drops.

Mix the ground ingredients; do likewise with the oils; then add the oil to the ground mixture gradually; keep stirring it for some time in order to have it thoroughly mixed.

JOCKEY CLUB SACHET POWDER.

This is one of the most popular powders, and will hold its place with any of them. This recipe may be relied upon for producing a first-class jockey club, and should be used when a very fine quality of lasting powder is wanted. Many ladies select this for filling sachet bags, or for putting in pillows and elsewhere.

Take
Pulverized Orris Root, 2 ounces.
Ground Vanilla Beans, 2 drachms.
"   Lavender Flowers, ½ ounce.
"   Orange Flowers, ½ ounce.
"   Pale Rose Flowers, ½ ounce.
True Musk Grain, 10 grains.
Pulv. Gum Benzoin, 3 drachms.
Oil Sandal Wood, 1 drachm.
"   Neroli, 10 drops.
"   Bergamot, 25 drops.
"   Civet, 20 drops.

Mix the ground ingredients with the powdered; mix the oils together and add them to the other mixture slowly; keep mixing it while the oils are being added, and stir up together until the whole is commingled.

VIOLET SACHET POWDER.

The following recipe will make a violet sachet powder which will compare with the most expensive; either domestic or imported.

All the ingredients, especially the flowers, must be fresh and of the best quality; otherwise the powder will fall short of its usual perfection.

Take

Ground Peony, ½ ounce.
   "   Violet Flowers (Odorata) ½ ounce.
   "   Lily of the Valley Flowers ½ ounce.
   "   Red Rose Leaves, 1 ounce.
   "   Flor. Orris Root, 3 ounces.
   "   Benzoic Acid, 1 drachm.
Pulv. Mace, 2 drachms.
Oil Bitter Almonds, 5 drops.
  " Ceylon Cinnamon, 10 drops.

Mix the ground ingredients with the powders; then add the oils and benzoic acid; then thoroughly rub together, and completely commingle.

LAVENDER SACHET POWDER.

This recipe makes a lavender powder that is not excelled by any; it is a peculiar odor; anybody who likes lavender must be very much pleased, as it has all the characteristic odor of it.

Take

Ground Lavender Flowers, 4 ounces.
"   Orange Flowers, sweet, ¼ ounce.
"   Red Rose Leaves, ½ ounce.
"   Rosemary flowers, ¼ ounce.

Pulv. Gum Benzoin, 2 drachms.
Gro. Tonka Beans, 2 drachms.
Oil Lavender Flowers, 3 drachms.
" Lemongrass, ½ drachm.

Prepare by mixing the ground ingredients with the powder; mix the oils and add them gradually to the other ingredients; rub together until all are thoroughly mixed.

PART X.

AROMATIC,

OR PRESTON SMELLING SALTS.

Many ladies use and carry with them when they go out, some kind of smelling salts ; especially in traveling. They use it as a preventive and cure of headache and faintness.

The recipe which follows makes a preparation much esteemed by those using it. I kept this and the next following preparation in stock when I carried on the drug business, and my patrons bought both kinds largely.

During an extended trip or absence from home, as no doubt many of my readers know by experience, it is sometimes worth more than ten times their cost to have

at hand smelling salts that you know to be good restoratives. The relief it will afford at such times can only
be appreciated by those who have experienced its beneficial influence. Do not travel without it if you are
subject to sudden attacks of faintness or headache.

PRESTON SMELLING SALTS.

NUMBER 1.

Take
Granulated Carbonate Potassa, 2 drachms.
" Muriate Ammonia, 2 drachms.
Pulv. Camphor Gum, 20 grains.
" Cubebs, 20 grains.
" Coriander Seed, 5 grains.
Oil Sassafras, 1 drop.
" Cloves, 2 drops.
" Peppermint, 2 drops.
" Bergamot, 2 drops.

To prepare this smelling salts, rub the carbonate
potassa and muriate ammonia together *lightly ;* then add
the camphor, cubebs and oils ; rub all together lightly,
yet enough to have all evenly divided. When completed it should be put in to a bottle and well corked up.
A glass stoppered, wide mouthed bottle is the best to
keep it in, where it cannot lose its strength.

Directions for use.

Inhale it from a pungent or smelling bottle. When
it has lost its strength it can be renewed by adding to
it a few drops of concentrated ammonia water; this
can be had at the drug store. Any kind of a bottle,
from which the vapor can be inhaled, will answer it
is well to be a little cautious in applying the bottle to

the nose, as it sometimes will give a severe shock if too much of it is inhaled at a time. Therefore, when you smell of the bottle, start in easy to see how strong it is.

SMELLING SALTS.

NUMBER 2.

This recipe will make an aromatic smelling salts that very closely resembles the best Preston salts. When it is kept well corked, it will retain its strength and medicinal properties for a long time. It will be observed that this powder becomes stronger after having been made some time, (provided it has been kept well corked). This is a peculiarity of the combination. If the amount the recipe calls for is too large, have a smaller quantity put up ; if too small have the quantity doubled, as desired.

Take

    Granulated Muriate Ammonia, ½ ounce.

        "   Carbonate Potassa, ½ ounce.

    Pulverized Orris-Root, 10 grains.

        "   Cubebs, 20 grains.

        "   Cinnamon, 20 grains.

        "   Cloves, 20 grains.

        "   Camphor Gum, 3 grains.

    Oil Sassafras, 2 drops.

    " Bergamot, 4 drops.

Prepare by mixing the ammonia and potassa with the powdered ingredients, add the oils, and rub all together until they are well mixed; always keep tightly corked when it is not in use.

This powder may be used just the same as the one preceding it, and for the same purposes.

PART XI.

GLOVE POWDER.

I believe I am justified in saying that ladies will appreciate this powder. For how well they all realize what an advantage it is to have something to dust into their kid gloves, that will at once overcome the difficulty of getting their gloves on; a matter that is at times very embarrassing, besides causing any amount of ill temper.

This powder will positively enable persons to draw their gloves on without the least trouble. It will save all annoyance and ruffling of temper, and be a positive aid in putting on the gloves. With this powder, it will be as easy as it is of slipping on a pair of mits, even in hot weather; so that ladies need not dread the ordeal.

It also prevents the excessive perspiration of the hands, which some are so much troubled with.

It can also be used with the same amount of satisfaction in cooling the surface of the skin when overheated. This recipe makes a preparation which it is truly a pleasure to use. It will be highly appreciated for its absorbent properties, in which respect it has no superior.

Take
Pulv. White Talc or White French Chalk, 6 ounces.
" Fuller's Earth, 2 ounces.
[This must be in the very finest powder.]
Oil Sandal Wood, ½ drachm.
" Neroli Petale, 10 drops.
" Rose Geranium, ½ drachm.

Oil Bitter Almonds, 4 drops.

True Grain Musk, 3 grains.

Prepare by mixing the powders; then add the oils; mix gradually; then add the musk, and mix all together very thoroughly.

Keep in bottle with wide mouth, or in box with a slide perforated top; keep the slide closed until wanted for use.

Directions for use.

Hold the kid gloves open, and dust the powder into them freely before putting them on. Some of the powder may also be rubbed on the hands and fingers. It may also be used in the shoes; dust it in the back some part where the heel comes in contact with the shoes; also put on inside of the instep, and on to the stockings, for excessive perspiration. Dust on the skin with puff or rub it on with the hands. In fact, it may be used in any way which is most convenient.

PART XII.

MISCELLANEOUS FORMULAS

OR

FAMILY RECIPES.

PREPARATIONS FOR CLEANING AND POLISHING.

The following are recipes for making preparations that are in daily demand. I trust they will prove as useful to my readers as they were to numbers of my former patrons, by whom they have been used with unqualified approbation.

They will be found perfectly reliable, practical, and effective, and will make first-class preparations, at about one half the cost that is usually charged for similar ones in the stores.

There are a great many so-called practical recipes published; but when brought to a test they generally lack practicability, or are found short in some things. This is only too true of a great many of the published formulas, which have actually no claim whatever to a place among recipes of worth.

They generally have been picked up at random, and have no substantial bottom to them. I abhor professionally and personally a deceptive and worthless recipe. It puts good ones in disrepute.

The nature of chemical combinations would not permit these fugitive recipes, as written, to be what is claimed for them; for this would be entirely out of the question. To verify my assertion, attempt to have one put up just as the recipe says, and see what the result will be.

I have had some of these reputed valuable recipes come to me to be compounded that I did not dare to put up, without amendment, as serious consequences would certainly have followed. But the recipes published in this volume have knowledge and experience back of them, so that they are perfectly reliable, practical and useful, and are the actual outgrowth of special study of the subject during nearly twenty years' experience as a druggist. I have had ample opportunity for trying and testing them. I therefore do not offer this work to the public filled up with a lot of stuff that nobody knows anything about, or which lacks the necessary substantial bottom.

The recipes and reading matter are plainly written; they can be understood by all and may be put up by anybody, without recourse to professional chemists or druggists, except for the materials.

DETERGENT CREAM.

This is a preparation for taking out grease and stains of all kinds. The composition will show that it can be used without in the least injuring the material or fabric to be cleaned. It can be used for taking out all kinds of stains. It is really a great preparation for cleaning up things. Many articles may be washed in it, as in ordinary washing. I do not mean that colored goods can be handled in this way, for it might take the color all out of them, but any thing which will bear ordinary washing can safely be cleaned with this cream.

Take
    Tincture Benzoin, plain, $\frac{1}{2}$ drachm.
    Pure White Castile Soap, 2 ounces.
    Hot Water, 3 pints.
    Pulverized Borax, 1 ounce.
    Aqua Ammonia, 2 ounces.
    Sulphuric Ether, 2 drachms.
    Glycerine, 1 ounce.
    Alcohol, 1 ounce.

Prepare this by cutting the soap up into small pieces; then dissolve it in the hot water; it may be heated, if necessary, to accomplish this. Then, while still hot, add the borax; when this is dissolved, allow the solution to become cold; then add the ammonia, glycerine, alcohol, benzoin, and ether ; shake or stir all together; then bottle. It should be agitated during the time it is being bottled, in order to have the ether well distributed. Keep well corked until wanted for use.

Directions for using.

Apply the cream to stains with soft sponge or soft cloth. If the goods will bear washing, wash them directly in the cream, as in suds. Then rinse off the article with clean water and allow it to dry nicely.

GREASE ERADICATOR.

This formula will make another preparation for taking out grease spots and stains of all kinds; it is very similar to the one preceding, yet it is different in a number of respects. Some people prefer it to the other ; I therefore concluded to insert them both, and give people their choice. They are both good, and will prove so on being used.

Take
  Castile Soap, 2 ounces.
  Bicarbonate Soda, 1 ounce.
  Pulverized Borax, 1 ounce.
  Carbonate Ammonia, 2 ounces.
  Alcohol, 2 ounces.
  Cologne, ½ ounce.
  Sulphuric Ether, ½ ounce.
  Boiling Water, 4 pints.

To prepare this, cut the soap into small pieces, by

shaving it; have the water boiling hot; put soap, borax, and ammonia in it; stir until they are all dissolved; allow the solution to get cold; then add the cologne and sulphuric ether to it; shake well, and bottle up for use as desired. Keep it tightly corked.

Directions.

This preparation may be used about the same as the previous one. Apply with sponge, or in any convenient way. Do not use it on fancy colors without trying a small piece of the goods to see if the color will stand.

FOR CLEANING KID GLOVES.

I have found that the following preparation will do this very nicely, perhaps better than a large number of preparations which are sold at high prices. It is very simple and inexpensive, and may be used freely.

Take
> Good quality Benzine, 2 pints.
> Chloroform, 1 drachm.
> Sulphuric Ether, 1 drachm.
> Cologne, 1 drachm.

Mix all together; keep in bottle well corked.

Directions for using.

The best way is to put the gloves on the hands; then take a small sponge; saturate it with the mixture and thoroughly clean the gloves; it should be put on all over the gloves. Repeat the application sufficiently to have the gloves come out bright and clean. Some colors must be carefully handled or the color will come off; try the preparation on the gloves in some place where it will not show if the color should come off. The gloves may also be washed in this in the ordinary way. Rub them between the fingers thoroughly until you have the stains and dirt all off; then hang them up to dry, after which they must be stretched. It is absolutely necessary to be cautious in using this. The benzine is very inflammable, and under no consideration should it be used anywhere near a fire or light; nor the gloves hung near the stove to dry. Serious accidents sometimes occur from the careless handling of benzine ; it can, however, be used with perfect safety when the above caution is observed.

LIQUID PREPARATION.

FOR CLEANING AND POLISHING SOLID AND PLATED WARE AND PLATE GLASS.

I am well aware that the market is full of preparations for this purpose ; and also that the dear public have to pay a good high price for the privilege of buying them, at least if they possess true merit.

I can further assure the public that with the recipe following can be made just as effective a preparation as any in the market at a very large percentage less cost; it will also be decidedly less injurious to the ware.

The ladies have to deal with this matter, and they know only too well how difficult it is to get a preparation which will perform the work and not injure the ware. I believe this preparation will produce satisfactory results ; such at least has been the experience of people who have used it.

12

Take
   Pure Precipitate Chalk, 3 ounces.
   Finely Pulverized Fuller's Earth, 2 drachms.
   Aqua Ammonia, 2 ounces.
   Alcohol, 2 ounces.
   Laundry Soap, ½ ounce.
   Water, 1 pint.

Prepare this by shaving the soap into small pieces; then procure a bottle holding over a pint, put the powders and soap into it; then pour on the ammonia and alcohol (these may be mixed before putting them in the bottle, as may also the powders); then pour on the water, and shake all up well, before using it.

Directions.

Always shake well before using the mixture; apply it to the article to be cleaned with sponge or soft cloth; it should be put on well and rubbed hard, to produce the best effect. Repeat the application as often as necessary to thoroughly clean the ware; use chamois skin or soft woollen cloth to complete the polish.

Plate glass must be washed in plain water first; then apply the mixture; rub it on hard; then finish by rinsing off, wiping with cloth; then rub with chamois skin or woollen cloth. If this is applied to the plate thoroughly there is nothing that can produce a finer polish.

———

POLISHING POWDER.

FOR CLEANING AND POLISHING SOLID AND PLATED WARE.

As some people prefer a preparation for cleaning and polishing their solid and plated ware in powder form, I will try to satisfy all by giving my recipes for making both the powder and liquid.

The polish powder is made as follows:

Take

Finely Pulverized Fuller's Earth, 4 ounces.
" " Rotten-stone, 4 ounces.
" " Drop Chalk, 4 ounces.

Rub the powders together thoroughly, it will then be ready to use; keep in a box.

Directions for using.

This powder may be applied to the article to be cleaned with a soft cloth, rubbing it hard until it is thoroughly cleaned; then finishing the polish by using a chamois skin until the desired lustre is obtained. The powder may also be moistened with water and applied with a sponge; put on the sponge some of the powder and apply it to the article to be cleaned; rub it on all over the surface until it looks clear and bright; then rinse off with clean water; wipe dry with soft cloth and finish the polish by rubbing briskly with soft chamois skin, until the desired lustre is obtained. The harder the article is rubbed, the more it will shine.

PREPARATION FOR CLEANING AND POLISHING BRASS AND COPPER WARE.

How to keep the brass and copper looking bright and clean greatly troubles many housekeepers. I have often heard them relate sad tales of tribulation in connection with this matter. Now this work can be done without much labor if you have the right thing to do it with.

If you have any brass or copper ware utensils or trimmings about the house or office which have become discolored or uncleanly the following mixture will restore them. It will take off all the discoloration or accumulation of matter, and the ware will come out clean and bright as new. It is really surprising to see the transformation that takes place on their being cleaned with this preparation.

After the articles have been thoroughly cleaned and brightly polished with this mixture, apply it to them occasionally in order to keep them bright, as new. This can be done very easily and quickly after the first hard cleaning. Try it and see.

Take
    Oxalic Acid, 2 ounces.
    Finely Pulv. Rotten-stone, 2 ounces.
    Hot Water, 1 pint.

Dissolve the oxalic acid in the hot water; then add the pulverized rotten-stone, and shake up well.

The bottle that this mixture is kept in should be labelled *Poison*, as the oxalic acid is poisonous.

The mixture should therefore be handled with caution; it should never be left standing where children can possibly get hold of it. It is always infinitely easier to guard against an accident than to remedy one after it has happened.

Directions for using.

Always shake the mixture well before using. It can be applied to the article to be cleaned with a sponge or cloth; it must be used freely and rubbed on very hard, especially if the article is discolored and tarnished. After being thoroughly cleaned until it looks bright, it should be well rinsed with clean water until you get off all of the mixture, (it is necessary to be particular about this every time the preparation is used); then wipe the article dry with cloth. When this is done, finish the polish by using either chamois skin or soft woollen cloth to complete the polish.

The fact that the above mixture contains oxalic acid, which is an active poison, does not in any way make it dangerous to use. I can assure my readers that there is not one bit of danger in using it when handled according to directions. There is nothing that will do this work so satisfactorily as this combination. I have used it myself, and seen it tried a great many times with entire success.

BLACK INK.

This is an article nearly everybody buys already made, because they do not want the bother of making it, or have no recipe for doing so. The following recipe is very simple, and makes a first class ink at considerably less cost than mercantile ink.

It will pay anybody who uses much ink to make it from this formula. It is scarcely any trouble to do it, the ink will keep any length of time, and does not become mouldy. I would suggest a trial of this ink; when properly made from pure material it makes an ink that will suit nearly everybody.

Take

Pure Black Analine, (*the kind called Nigrosin*), 2 drachms.

Oil Cloves, 2 drops.

Pure Carbolic Acid, 2 grains.
Pulv. gum Arabic, ½ drachm.
Soft water, 6 ounces.

Prepare the ink as follows:

Heat the water boiling hot; then pour it into a half pint bottle (the bottle should of course be previously warmed in order to prevent its breaking when the hot water is poured into it). The Nigrosin should then be added to the water, and well shaken until it is dissolved. After it is cold, add the oil, cloves, carbolic acid, and gum arabic. Shake the whole together until thoroughly mixed; it will then be ready to use. The above amount can of course be increased to a pint if desired, by simply doubling up the materials.

CARMINE INK.

The following recipe will make a first class red ink. It may be used for all purposes. There is no red or carmine ink in the market that is superior to this one. It is easy to make and inexpensive. Whenever you desire to use a red ink have this recipe made up. It will prove very satisfactory.

Take
    Pure Carmine, (No. 40) 1 drachm.
    Aqua Ammonia, 2 drachms.
    Mucilage Acacia, 1 drachm.
    Rose Water, 6 drachms.

Dissolve the carmine in the ammonia; then add the rose water and mucilage; shake well together; keep well corked (rubber cork is the best for this), or else have a glass stoppered bottle.

INDELIBLE INK
FOR MARKING WHITE CLOTHES.

Take
Nitrate Silver Crystals, 2 drachms.
Pure water, 5 drachms.
Mucilage Acacia, 1 drachm.
Concentrated Water Ammonia, 2 drachms.

To prepare the Indelible Ink—
Dissolve the nitrate silver in the pure water; then add the concentrated water ammonia, and shake the mixture lightly. If the ammonia don't completely redissolve the precipitate which forms, add a little more to it. When the solution has been nicely accomplished, then add the mucilage and shake all together. It will then be ready to use. It is a good plan to cover the bottle with blue paper and keep the ink in a dark place, as exposure to light will decompose the combination; it will thereby become deteriorated, and in a short time unfit to use. This is also true of all good indelible inks.

Directions.

This ink can be used with an ordinary steel, or any other pen; it must, however, be perfectly clean.

The goods to be marked should contain no starch, as the ink will not take so well on starch. Open out the garment upon an even and perfectly smooth table; then smooth all the folds out of the cloth, where the marking is to be done; then write whatever you wish on the piece just the same as you would if you were writing on paper.

Expose the place on which the marking has been done to the rays of the sun or to the heat of a stove; cr, after the ink is dry, run a hot flat-iron over the place.

The heating of the marked spot will at once bring out the ink, plain, bold, and permanent. The heat may be applied in any way that may be convenient, but the heat is what makes the ink stay in good.

If the above directions are carried out, you will find your marking will stay; which is not the case with some inks.

Of course this recipe must be put up just right, when the combination is properly put together and the ink is correctly handled and applied, there will be no failure in getting good results.

INK REMOVER.

It is frequently a matter of considerable advantage to know what will remove ink stains. No doubt many of my readers have had personal experience with this very matter.

Note.— The following preparation will remove the stains or spots left by anything but indelible ink. If it is used on colored goods great care should be exercised, in order not to disturb the colors, as many of the fancy colors are very easily affected by the application of chemicals.

To remove ink or other stains from carpets or colored goods of any kind, great caution should be used in applying any preparation, to prevent some valuable fabric from being ruined.

The following preparation can be used on some kinds of colors without disturbing them. I would, however suggest, for safety to those using it on colored goods, to try it on some part where it would not show if it should take the color out; then act according to what the trial proves. It may be used upon all white goods without the least danger, as it will in no way injure the goods.

It is also an extraordinary preparation for bleaching clothes and for a washing fluid. To make this—

Take
   Fresh Chlorinated, or, as it is called, Chloride of, Lime, ¼ pound.
   Washing Soda, 1 pound.
   Water, 1 quart.

Prepare by putting washing soda in water, and boil until it is dissolved; then add the chloride of lime, and keep it hot until all is dissolved; when cold strain and keep in bottle for use.

When wanted for bleaching, or to use as washing fluid, it can be made to order, or kept ready, in large quantity, in crocks or jars, covered up tightly. It is very much liked as an aid in washing clothes. It brings them out a beautiful white. It must not be used too strong. Put a small quantity in each water, but more in the blueing water that the clothes are soaked in. When it is wanted for removing ink stains, and you have none made up, buy some solution of chlorinated soda (which is the same thing), and use it.

Directions for taking out ink.

Apply the solution to the spot or stain quite freely; allow it to remain on a short time; then take it up on a sponge or cloth, and rinse the spot off with clean water several times, in order to get the solution all out; then dry it well. If the spot is still there, repeat the

operation as many times as necessary to take it out. Be
sure to rinse the goods well with clean water each time.
If the stains are on white goods, it may be used as above,
or the place where the stains or spots are may be washed
in the solution, or allowed to soak in it a short time;
then rubbed between the fingers. This may, if necessary, be repeated several times; then thoroughly rinse
with clear water, and hang up to dry where it will dry
slow.

When the solution is used for bleaching, place the
goods in enough of the preparation to cover them;
allow to remain, with an occasional stirring, until they
have bleached nicely; then rinse thoroughly in several
different lots of clear water. Then, if it is the right
time of year, and it is convenient, lay on the grass to
dry: otherwise, hang them up to dry.

This preparation has been used a long time for bleaching, and has always proved perfectly satisfactory.

The goods should not be left in too long; an unrea-
sonable time might affect the cloth.

WASHING FLUID.

This recipe produces a preparation that makes washing comparatively easy, and, properly used, it in no way
injures the clothes. It materially reduces the labor of
washing; saves soap, fuel and time—all very important
factors in every-day life.

Take
    Salts of Tartar, 1 ounce.
    Pulverized Muriate Ammonia, 1 ounce.

Pulverized Borax, 1½ ounce.
Concentrated Potash, 1 pound.
Water, 1 gallon.

Prepare by heating the water hot; then put all the other ingredients in, and let them dissolve; it may be stirred with a stick occasionally until they dissolve. Keep it covered up when not stirring it. When it is cold, it may be put up in bottles, or in something which can be tightly covered or corked, and allowed to remain so until wanted for use.

This makes a strong, caustic preparation, and should never be kept where children can get at it; possibly they might get into it and do themselves considerable injury. The surest way with children is to keep all such things out of their reach.

Directions.

The washing fluid may be used by putting a quantity of it into the water, in which the clothes should stand, soaking over night; there must be enough water to cover them, and enough of the fluid used to have the desired effect. This depends largely on conditions; where the clothes are real dirty, more will have to be used than if they were not soiled much. Some of the fluid may also be put into the rest of the water; all except the blueing water. A few trials will show you just what quantity to use; half or even less of the amount of the recipe may be used if the whole proves too strong.

RUST REMOVER.

This is another thing well worth knowing; for, at times, it will be valuable knowledge to possess. How often do linen goods become stained with iron rust, which has to stay on them, simply because people do not know how to remove it. I have found that the combination made from the recipe following will remove it very easily. I put this well-tried recipe in this book for the benefit of those who may be in want of just its kind of a preparation. It should only be used on white goods.

Take

Pulverized Citric Acid, ½ ounce.
"   Oxalic Acid, ½ ounce.

Mix them together and keep in a perfectly dry bottle. It should always be kept well corked, and marked or labelled POISON.

Directions.

The stained spot should be wet with clean water; then sprinkle some of the powder on the stain or iron rust, and allow it to remain there some time; then rinse with clear water. If the spot or stain has disappeared, then rinse again several times; if, however, the spot still appears, wet the spot and sprinkle on some of the powder; allow it to remain for a short time; then wash off and rinse with clear water several times, until the spot and stains have been entirely removed.

FURNITURE POLISH.

The following formulas are for making preparations to use upon furniture, which has become marred by use. How often we see furniture that looks as though it has had some experience with a cyclone. These preparations will renew the finish on all kinds of furniture and cabinet ware, making old furniture to look like new. It is actually surprising to see what a change takes place in the appearance of any old piece of furniture after being treated with this preparation. If you have cabinet ware that requires a little rejuvenating try what can be done with this polish.

FURNITURE POLISH.

NUMBER ONE.

Take
  Boiled Oil, 8 ounces.
  Raw Linseed Oil, 12 ounces.
  Turpentine, 8 ounces.
  Benzine, 4 ounces.
  Acetic Acid, 2 ounces.
  Oil Sassafras, 2 drachms.
Mix all together and shake up well.

Directions.

These different furniture polishes are all to be used in the same way. Shake the mixture hard, and then apply to the article to be polished with an old soft woollen cloth; woollen is the best. Do not put on too much, but apply it all over; after this has been done thoroughly, take another soft cloth, and finish up by rubbing very hard and brisk until the surface appears newly polished. The harder it is rubbed the brighter the finish will appear. The furniture may be treated with the polish just as often as it may be necessary in order to keep it in good condition. This depends, of course, on how the furniture is used.

I have added numbers two and three, so that my readers can take their choice of three excellent preparations.

FURNITURE POLISH.

NUMBER TWO.

Take

    Boiled Oil, ½ pint.

    Common Vinegar, ½ pint.

    Butter of Antimony, 2 drachms.

    Oil Cloves, 1 drachm.

Mix all together.

Shake well and use as suggested in preceding directions.

FURNITURE POLISH.

NUMBER THREE.

Take

    Raw Linseed Oil, ½ pint.

    Boiled Linseed Oil, ½ pint.

    Alcohol, 4 ounces.

    Cider Vinegar, 4 ounces.

    Turpentine, 8 ounces.

    Red Analine, 10 grains.

    Oil Wintergreen, 2 drachms.

Prepare this by dissolving the red analine in the alcohol; add the vinegar to the boiled oil, and shake up well; then mix all the ingredients together and shake the whole very thoroughly.

This can be used on any kind of finish or furniture. Use same as directed under preceding recipe.

MUCILAGE.

This is something that most people use more or less; it can be made just as well as to buy it, in large or small quantities. This recipe will produce a first-class mucilage. The sticky quality cannot be excelled; it will also keep well. It is good for any purpose that a mucilage is wanted.

Take
Gum Arabic, 2 ounces.
  Dextrine, ½ ounce.
  Oil Cloves, 2 drops.
  " Sassafras, 2 drops.
  Carbolic Acid, 2 grains.
  Water, 4 ounces.

Prepare by dissolving the gum arabic and dextrine in the water. Hot water will hasten solution; cold water will dissolve it, but takes longer. It should be stirred occasionally during the time it is dissolving.

When dissolved add the carbolic acid and oils to the solution; shake or stir well together. Then strain it if it should be somewhat dirty. When first quality of gum arabic is used there will be no need of straining it. Use with brush, same as any mucilage.

MOTH DESTROYER.

This will very much interest all housekeepers. There is probably nothing in household matters which is more troublesome to contend with than moths; and carpet bugs are nearly as bad. At times they have the pper hand, and it seems almost impossible to get rid

of them. They try the patience of many a good house-
keeper, and the question is asked again and again, how
can we get rid of them. When appealed to for help, I
have put up the preparation made from the following
recipe, and it always worked perfectly if the instructions were carefully followed. It is necessary to use
the preparation faithfully until all the pests have been
destroyed or driven away.

I have seen its effects many times and consequently
have no hesitation in suggesting its use, I feel confident that after you use it you will be as well pleased
with the results as others have been, and be willing to
incur several times its cost rather than go without it.
Those who possess this book will have the benefit, at
little cost, of valuable information on his and innumerable other subjects.

Take
  Pure Carbolic Acid, ½ ounce.
  Oil Cloves, ½ ounce.
  Oil of Cedar Wood, 2 ounces.
  Camphor Gum, 3 ounces.
  Pure Alcohol, 1 pint.
Prepare by dissolving the camphor gum in the alco-
hol; then add the oils and carbolic acid. Shake well
together and keep corked until it is wanted. One pint
of turpentine may be added to make it cheaper.

Directions.

When used for carpets, it should be applied to the
floor when the carpets are to be tacked down, and also
to the edge of the carpets. This must be done very
thoroughly. If there are any crevices, they too
must be well saturated with the Destroyer. This

can perhaps be done to the best advantage by the use of a feather, dipping it in the liquid, then applying to every part of the crevice; you can use a small soft brush in same way.

Another important matter is this: the edge of the carpets where they are tacked down or under, should be thoroughly overhauled occasionally. It is a good plan to give the edges of the carpet a thorough sweeping with a good stiff broom at least once or twice a week; this will have a tendency to break up the nests, and prevent breeding; and enable you by the use of the preceding preparation to annihilate the moths and carpet bugs. It should be remembered that these insects seek dark and secluded corners and the back of furniture where the broom seldom reaches ; here is just where they make their homes, and these dark places must be often stirred up, so that when you use your preparations you will be able to reach them. I am satisfied, from looking into this matter, that these insects may be controlled without a great amount of trouble if it is only seen to in time, "An ounce of prevention is worth a pound of cure," and so it is in this matter ; by a proper course in the premises there will be no need whatever of your having any moths or carpet bugs in the house. If the above suggestions are followed and the Destroyer is regularly used, I undertake to say there will be an end to the moth promptly in your household. Do not tack the carpet with a large number of tacks. Put one in only here and there ; you can then apply the Destroyer without any difficulty, and besides you can readily sweep about the edges of the carpet and corners of the floor. This would be a step in the right direction. After the carpet has once been put down and tacked, and allowed to remain a short time, it will keep its place even though two thirds of the tacks are withdrawn. There will be no difficulty whatever in keeping clear of these troublesome pests if eternal vigilance is exercised. Use the Destroyer on other goods, such as furs, clothing, and anything the bugs infest, substantially in the same manner. The best way is to use an atomizer for treating the various things which you desire to protect from the pest, aside from carpets on the floor, spray thoroughly with the atomizer, so that the mist will cover, without wetting them in any place. Furniture of all kinds can be treated in this way better, perhaps, than in any other. Of course it may be used in any other way, such as saturating either paper or cloth and wrapping it up in the article; or by sprinkling the articles lightly.

"THE BUFFALO OR CARPET BUG."

How to keep a house clear of these troublesome pests, and how to free the premises after they once get in, is one of the most difficult problems housekeepers have to contend with.

The Buffalo Bug, commonly called the Carpet Bug, seems to thrive wherever it obtains a foothold. Its work of destruction is not confined to carpets, but on the contrary it attacks anything which has the smallest amount of wool in its composition. Wool seems to be their favorite matter. On this diet they not only thrive

and grow fat, but also multiply amazingly fast; they
are therefore able to do an extraordinary amount of
damage—destroying valuable garments and wearing
apparel in an exceedingly short space of time. These
dreaded little pests always appear to be hungry,
and to satisfy their ferocious appetites, do not hesitate
to attack and take up anything that happens to be in
their reach. Cotton, or any other clothing or cloth
which they come in contact with has to succumb to
their onslaught.

I can truly say, from experience, that the price of
the destruction and extermination of these hairy little
pests, must be "eternal vigilance." If housekeepers
would keep up a perpetual war on this bug, their houses
would not be infested with it, and they would not have
valuable carpets, clothing and other things destroyed
by its ravages.

There is nothing more effective in preventing its
gaining an entrance than frequent and thorough airing
of all articles that are liable to their attacks. It is necessary to expose such articles to the rays of the sun frequent-
quently. Do not keep them shut up in dark places,
for it is in such places that the bugs find plenty of time
and materials upon which to begin their work of silent
destruction.

I do not put it too strong when I say they must be
fought with a strong will and frequently with strong
weapons; for though they are little pests, how mighty
and great are their works! They not only destroy
valuable goods, but the misery and unhappiness they
cause in some households is pitiable to behold. If any
of my readers think this pen picture is too strongly

drawn, I respectfully ask them to place themselves back of a drug counter for a few months, where the trials of the housewife have to be listened to.

The following recipe makes a combination which will positively prove a boon to all who have contended in vain with the dreaded little hairy fellows called Carpet Bugs. This is not one of those humbug preparations for which the false claim is made that they will exterminate the bugs. It has been tried a great many times, and has never proved a failure when properly used. Try it.

Take
　　Fine Table Salt, 1 pound.
　　Pure Insect Powder, ½ pound.
　　Pulv. Borax, ½ pound.
　　　" 　Yellow Sandal Wood, 2 ounces.

Mix the powders together thoroughly, and keep tightly covered in bottles.

Directions for using.

When the powder is wanted for carpets on the floor, use it freely by sprinkling a layer close to the base board. If there is any space between the floor and base board, fill a small bellows with the powder; then blow the powder into the space as far as it will go ; also blow a liberal amount into all the spaces and crevices that are infested.

When this plan is carried out carefully and thoroughly, the results will be very satisfactory.

This powder may also be used to good advantage as a preventive. "An ounce of prevention is worth a pound of cure."

If carpets or other goods are to be laid away, do not

fail to treat them first with this powder, or one of the moth destroyers made after my recipes.

This powder is also very effective in preventing roaches and water bugs from gaining an entrance into a house, as well as for exterminating them. Sprinkle it around freely; blow it into the crevices and spaces, especially around the water pipes. This should be done frequently until the premises are free from them.

You may rest assured, if the work is done faithfully, the reward will be the certain and total extermination of the nests.

SUMMER DRINKS.

There are thousands of people who would like to make a pleasant, light, healthy, cooling drink for the summer season.

Of course there are no end of preparations of this character which are now sold, nor of recipes for making them; but there are very few among them all which meet the requirements; they are all lacking in some feature, besides being inconvenient and generally expensive to buy.

The following recipes will produce preparations of this character equal to any which can be made at home or wherever a person may be spending the summer season, with little trouble and expense.

It will positively pay anybody having a liking for these agreeable, health-giving and cooling summer drinks, to make them after these recipes.

GINGER ALE OR BEER.

Make as follows :—Take

    Granulated Sugar, 1 pound.
    Ground Ginger Root, 3 ounces.
    Pure Cream Tartar, 1 ounce.
    The juice of two lemons.
    The whites of two eggs.
    Boiling water, 1 gallon.

Prepare as follows:

Add the sugar to the boiling water; then add the ground ginger root and cream tartar; cover up and keep hot 15 minutes; then stir it up well and allow it to get nearly cold; now strain it; then add the lemon juice (the lemons must be fresh and not bitter) and 1-2 pint best yeast; mix all up well by stirring; then allow it to remain standing from twelve to twenty-four hours, according to temperature, to start fermentation. When this has been done add the whites of the eggs (which should be beaten to a silvery froth) to the liquid; then bottle; keep in a cool place and use as desired.

When a nice quality of yeast can be secured, the eggs may be added before the yeast; then shake together and allow to stand twelve to twenty-four hours, when it may be poured off and the yeast added to the clear sparkling liquid; shake well and allow to stand a few hours in moderately warm place; then bottle as above.

SPRUCE BEER.

The following recipe produces what is generally called the Beer of Health by people that desire a cooling, health-giving, refreshing, mild summer drink. There is perhaps nothing made which will answer the purpose better than this preparation.

It can be used freely without any ill effects; it is actually a healthy drink; one in which the temperance as well as temperate people will find solace. It is a drink in which all may join, and quench their thirst to their heart's content. It will comfort the millions who must have something to help them tide over the hot season.

This recipe for making the Spruce Beer can be relied upon to make an article far superior to a great many of the preparations sold as Spruce Beer. Try it.

Take

Fresh Hops, *best quality*, 6 drachms.
    "   Ground Sassafras bark, 2 drachms.
Granulated Sugar, 1 pound.
Essence Spruce, 2 drachms.
    "   Allspice, 2 drachms.
Extract Jamaica Ginger, 2 drachms.
The whites of two eggs.
Boiling water, 1 gallon.

Prepare by adding the sugar, hops, and sassafras bark to the boiling water; stir well; cover up; let it stand twenty-four hours; then strain it through cloth; then add the essence of spruce, allspice and extract of ginger; then shake or stir up well, after which add half pint best yeast; let it stand from twelve to twenty-four hours; pour off the clear liquid, and add the whites of the two eggs, (which should be well beaten); shake together well and bottle for future use. Keep in cool place.

In making either of the preceding beers it may at times be necessary to change the proportions of the ingredients, or at least of some of them (in order to suit the taste). This can always be done : nobody need follow these recipes strictly. If you prepare the preparation just as here directed and it fails to suit the taste, change it by leaving out or adding, or reducing by water.

In selecting the yeast be sure the quality is good ; *yeast cakes* may be used, providing, of course, that they are of good quality.

In straining the beer be particular to get it clear; this affects its appearance very much, and, as is perhaps well known, a perfectly clear drink has a better taste and certainly is more appreciated by people that are fastidious and particular as to what they drink.

PART XIII.

External Medicinal Applications.

LINIMENTS.

These preparations are used a great deal for various purposes. I can positively say that the following recipes will produce preparations which will do anything that the highly advertised liniments will do. They will effect a cure of any kind whatever that can be done by any of the preparations in the market. Do not put any faith in the extravagant boast that the proprietary liniments alone will afford relief and effect a cure. When the effects of a good, strong, penetrating liniment are desired for soreness, lameness, pains, bruises, or for anything that an external application will alleviate or cure, do not hesitate to have one of these recipes put up. The liniment will positively afford relief when any remedy of this nature can give it.

For a general family liniment try the following:

"PAIN ANNIHILATOR"

NUMBER ONE.

Take
  Oil Origanum, ½ ounce.
  " Hemlock, ½ ounce.
  " Sassafras, ¼ ounce.
  Aqua Ammonia, ½ ounce.
  Laudanum, ½ ounce.
  Camphor Gum, 1 ounce.
  Tincture Cayenne Pepper, ¼ ounce.
  "   Arnica, 1 ounce.
  Pure Chloroform, ½ ounce.
  " Alcohol, ¾ pint.

Dissolve the camphor in the alcohol; add the oils and other ingredients; shake all well together. Keep well corked.

Directions.

Apply to parts affected, from two to four times a day. Rub it in with the hand thoroughly, or it may be applied to the parts with a cloth, then bandaged lightly, and keep the cloth well saturated with the liniment.

This makes a strong and sharp liniment; do not use it so freely as to blister the parts; this probably would do no harm, but might inconvenience a person considerably. Apply a small quantity often, and rub in well.

"PAIN ANNIHILATOR"

NUMBER TWO.

This recipe will also produce a very good liniment, to be used in same way as the preceding one.

Any of these liniments can be used with equally as satisfactory results upon horses or other animals as upon human beings. Remedies of this character are very often necessary for animals. I desire it to be thoroughly understood that at any time a good first-class liniment is wanted the following will not disappoint you. It is really a capital one for pain or aches of all kinds.

Take
Oil Wormwood, ¼ ounce.
" Sassafras, ½ ounce.
" Cocoanut, ¼ ounce.
" Peppermint, ⅛ ounce.
" Origanum, 1 ounce.
" Cedar, ½ ounce.
" Wintergreen, ¼ ounce.
Castor Oil, ½ ounce.
Sulphuric Ether, ½ ounce.
Alcohol, 1 pint.

Mix all together and shake well; keep the bottle corked.

Directions.

Apply to the affected parts from one to four times a day, as may be necessary. Rub on with the hand, or apply on cloth; or, after rubbing, bandage with cloth wet in the liniment.

RHEUMATIC LINIMENT.

How many suffer with that most troublesome malady—rheumatism?

This Rheumatic Liniment has cured a great many people who had suffered with this complaint, even after all kinds of remedies had been tried and all proved a failure. If an external application can be of any possible benefit this remedy is the one to use. But there are cases where internal treatment only is allowable. In fact there are at times conditions in connection with this complaint where the use of external remedies should under no consideration be sanctioned, as they might bring on dangerous consequences, and the case should be given in the charge of a reputable physician. But the cases are few in which there would be danger in using this liniment. It will cure most cases of rheumatism, neuralgia, lameness, stiff joints and all other ailments of that nature.

The oils and other ingredients should all be of the best quality and strictly fresh.

Liniment for General Use.

Take
  Oil Hemlock, ¼ ounce.
  " Cedar, ¼ ounce.
  " Juniper Berry, ½ ounce.

Oil Spearmint, ⅛ ounce.
" Wormwood, ⅛ ounce.
" Origanum, ¼ ounce.
Laudanum, ½ ounce.
Volatile Liniment, 1 ounce.
Alcohol, enough to make ½ pint.
Mix all together; keep well corked.

Directions.

Shake well each time and apply to the parts affected; rub on thoroughly from one to four times a day.

COMPOUND CAMPHOR LINIMENT.

This recipe will make a very strong and actively penetrating liniment, and gives immediate relief, and often cures aches and pains of all kinds to which liniments are adapted for either man or beast.

Take
Gum Camphor, 1 ounce.
Oil Origanum, 1 ounce.
" Sassafras, 1 drachm.
" Peppermint, 1 drachm.
Sweet Oil, 2 ounces.
Aqua Ammonia, ½ ounce.
Extract Jamaica Ginger, 1 ounce.
Alcohol, ¾ pint.

Dissolve the camphor in the alcohol; then add the other ingredients. Shake together and keep well corked.

Directions.

Apply to the affected parts from two to four times a day, rubbing it on hard each time; or it may be applied, then bandaged with cloth.

PART XIV.

OINTMENTS OR SALVES.

The following recipes are a few of my best for making these preparations. They are intended for everything that salves or ointments will cure or alleviate. I have endeavored to select my best recipes in order to make a work that will be of great benefit to those having occasion to use an ointment. To all such the following recipes will prove of great service in curing sores, cuts, bruises, aches, swellings and relieving pain. A great many of the proprietary ointments so extensively and persistently kept before the public cannot compare with the preparations which may be made after the following recipes:

To make a good

ALL-HEALING OINTMENT,

OR CURE-ALL SALVE.

Take

Clean Common Resin, 3½ ounces.
Yellow Beeswax, 1½ ounce.
Burgundy Pitch, ½ ounce.
Pure Fresh Lard, 4 ounces.
Oil Rosemary, 2 drachms.
" Sassafras, 2 drachms.
" Peppermint, 2 drachms.
Balsam Fir, 2 drachms.
Oil Hemlock, 1¼ drachm.
Pulv. Camphor, ½ drachm.

To prepare the ointment:

Take a small tin basin; set it on the stove; put in

the resin, beeswax and Burgundy pitch; heat them slowly until melted; then add the lard, allowing all to melt by slow heat. Then take the basin from the stove, and when nearly cold stir in the oils, balsam of fir and camphor gum; these may all be mixed together previous to adding them to the melted ingredients. Continue the stirring briskly until the mixture becomes so stiff that it will not separate; then put in wide mouthed bottles or jars before it gets too cold and stiff. Cork or cover these tightly.

If the wax, lard, pitch and resin should get too stiff to allow the oils and other ingredients to be stirred in well, the mixture must be warmed again.

The efficacy of the ointment depends considerably upon its being manipulated carefully; when this is done the result is a nicely finished and highly beneficial combination.

Directions.

It may be applied to the affected parts directly, or put on cloth and then applied.

COMPOUND TAR OINTMENT.

This recipe will make an extra good salve for healing and curing all kinds of sores; it is very cleansing, and is therefore especially adapted to the cure of long-standing sores, over which it seems to exercise an extraordinary healing power. For remarkable healing and curative properties, I can safely say it is not excelled by any salve in the market.

Take
> Simple Ointment, 1½ ounces.
> Pure Petrolatum, or Cosmoline, 1 ounce.
> Resin Cerate, ½ ounce.
> Pulverized Oxide Zinc, 2½ drachms.
> Oil Tar, 1 drachm.
> " Wintergreen, ½ drachm.
> " Cedar, ½ drachm.
> Pure Carbolic Acid, 1 drachm.
> Pulverized Boracic Acid, ½ drachm.

Mix all the oils with the carbolic acid ; then mix all of the ingredients together very thoroughly. When completed, it must be smooth and even. The simple ointment, petrolatum and resin cerate may be mixed together ; then add the boracic acid and oxide of zinc in small quantities until it is fairly well mixed ; then add the mixed oils, and complete the mixing by thorough and hard rubbing, until a fine smooth ointment is brought out.

Directions for using.

Apply to the affected parts, either directly or on cloth ; in either event the sore (if it be such) should always be protected by a covering of cloth. The dressing should be changed at least once a day, and the sore thoroughly cleansed. If it is a fresh cut, it should not be disturbed after the first dressing (which should be a good one) for several days, or until it can be done without again opening the cut; this will give it a chance to grow together. The treatment in its details must be governed by circumstances. When it is found necessary to employ these preparations, exercise your judgment in regard to their use.

THE J. A. B. OINTMENT.

This recipe is for making a good healing and curing salve for cuts, burns, sores, swellings, and the numerous other things for which ointments are used. It will surely produce an excellent salve for general use; it is very soothing, cleansing and healing. It is also an extra good salve for the various skin diseases.

Take

Resin Cerate, 2 ounces.
Plain Cosmoline, 2 "
Oil Cade, 1 drachm.
 " Sassafras, 1 drachm.
 " Peppermint, ½ drachm.
 " Wormwood, 1   "
 " Bergamot, ½   "
Balsam Peru, ½   "
 " Fir, 2 drachms.
Pure Carbolic Acid in Crystals, 1½ drachm.
Pulverized Sub-nitrate Bismuth, 4 drachms.

Mix the cosmoline and resin cerate; mix the oils and balsams, and add thereto the mixed cerate and cosmoline; then add the sub-nitrate bismuth, and thoroughly incorporate it; then add the carbolic acid, and continue stirring and mixing until the whole is incorporated together, when it will be a nice smooth ointment, ready to use. Keep it in a jar or wide-mouthed bottle, well corked; set it in a cool place until wanted for use.

Directions for using.

Apply this ointment to cuts, burns, scalds, and sores of all kinds; pains, swellings, and all the other ailments requiring a good ointment, either direct to the affected part, or on cloth, from one to two times a day. It is necessary to keep the sore thoroughly cleansed, especially in treating old sores, or open sores of any kind. In fresh cuts of wounds it may be necessary not to disturb the dressing for the first few days, when the dressing should be changed and everything freshened up. A successful cure will be speedily accomplished with careful attention to cleanliness and changing the bandage at least once a day on old or open wounds.

HEMORRHOID OINTMENT.

There is probably no affliction from which a great many people suffer such untold distress and misery as they do from hemorrhoids.

I have frequently been called upon by my patrons to put up something for the relief and cure of this most distressing malady.

The very nature of the complaint precludes a great many people from procuring relief. Consequently they continue to suffer untold torture.

The following recipe will produce a preparation which I assure my readers who may be suffering with this ailment, will come to them like the good Samaritan. Back of the drug counter I came in contact with a great deal that excited my sympathy, and have often felt that the relief of human suffering has its own reward. The timid and shrinking natures that will not seek relief from the source whence it is ordinarily obtained, can, with this book, have the means of procuring a mitigation of this disorder.

It would be very chimerical for me to say this preparation will cure everybody, because that cannot be done with any one treatment, as the conditions vary much in different cases.

But I can truthfully say that this ointment has afforded immediate relief, and eventually effected a cure of a good many cases. It is worth a trial by those suffering with this complaint.

Take
    Simple Ointment, 1 ounce.
    Benzoated Lard, 1   "
    Pulverized Nut Galls, ½ ounce.
    Citrine Ointment, ¼ ounce.
    Oil Fireweed, 1 drachm.
    " Sassafras, 10 drops.
    Pulverized Opium, ½ drachm.
    "   Menthol Crystals, 2 grains.
    "   Sub-nitrate Bismuth, 3 drachms.

Mix the simple ointment with the benzoated lard and citrine ointment; then rub the powders all together, and add them gradually to the other mixture; keep stirring the mixture until they are all nicely incorporated and the ointment is perfectly smooth and even. Keep in box or jar, well covered.

Directions for using.

This ointment must be applied to the rectum, and, if necessary, it should be carried up inside the rectum to reach the seat of trouble. This can be done by simply using the finger to apply it, or it may be placed there by the use of a syringe which is made specially for applying ointments and salves to piles or hemorrhoids.

It should be applied once or twice a day until relief is procured or a cure is effected. Frequently the condition of the bowels becomes a strong factor in the relief and cure of hemorrhoids, and it is very essential to have the bowels in a normal condition during the treatment of this organic trouble, and afterwards to keep them so.

PART XV.

MEDICAL RECIPES.

REMEDIES.

Under this head will be found recipes for making remedies, which will no doubt frequently save sending for a physician.   I here place in your hands remedies that will, when used in time, often prevent a siege of suffering, and also 'a doctor's bill.   In order to make this work still more worthy the approval of the public, I concluded to give my readers the benefit of the knowledge I possess in relation to various diseases and their remedies.   These prescriptions are thoroughly reliable; they are compositions that I have been in the habit of putting up for people when they came into the store and desired the benefit of my experience, and I have sold these preparations over the drug counter for a good many years, with happy results.

I desire to impress my readers with the fact that the formulas or prescriptions in this book are not to be classed among the hundreds of so-called recipes, for making all kinds of nostrums, that have been published and widely circulated.

The following are mostly my private recipes, or formulas, for making preparations which I have sold to my patrons for a number of years. I spent a great deal of time and thought in perfecting them, during nearly twenty years' active work in the drug business, most of which time was spent in Rochester, N. Y. During part of this time I gave my special thought to the matter in this work, with the expectation of some day placing it before the public.

REMEDY FOR BURNS.

How often is a remedy for burns or scalds wanted in an emergency or accident, when people have nothing effectual to use?

It is an extremely wise thing to know what to use in an emergency, when a child has been nearly burned or scalded to death, or a grown person has met with a similar accident.

I have been hurriedly called upon many times on just such occasions, to furnish relief for severe burns and scalds. The remedy which I invariably furnished for this purpose is actually very simple, and I have yet to see a case where, if used properly, it did not immediately prove beneficial. If at any time the reader should be called upon in such an emergency, I hope he will have ready the following infallible alleviator :

Take

Raw Linseed Oil, ½ pint.

Lime Water, ½ pint.

Mix together, by thoroughly shaking until it becomes milky and creamy ; it will then be ready to use.

Directions for using.

It should be applied to the burn immediately. Put on enough to cover up the surface of the injury, then wrap the affected part in cotton. When the burn or scald is of a nature that precludes this, apply the mixture to the surface, then cover with cotton well saturated with the mixture. After the saturated cotton has been applied to the injury, it should be covered with another layer of dry cotton ; this last layer should be thin, and the first one thick. Then the mixture must be applied at short intervals, in sufficient quantity to cover the injury ; this should always be put right on to the first layer of cotton.

If the case is very severe, take advantage of the above treatment while the doctor is on the way; or rather, use this mixture at once, then send for the doctor if necessary. The treatment should be continued until the injury is healed, unless it becomes necessary to apply some healing salve ; when such is the case, use one of my healing salves from previous pages.

EAR-ACHE REMEDY.

This most distressing ailment can usually be relieved or cured with the remedy made after the following recipe. It seldom fails to relieve the most excruciating pain. I do not claim that it will cure all cases—there are some that require different treatment—but it will almost invariably give relief, and that is a great thing when a person is suffering such terrible pain.

For the ear-ache, take—
Pure Glycerine, 3 drachms.
Laudanum, 1 drachm.
Mix together.

Directions.

This remedy may be used by dropping from one to four drops into the affected ear one to three times a day. It may also be applied by inserting in the ear a small piece of cotton with a few drops of the remedy on it.

It may be used for children as well as for adults.

If the remedy is dropped into the ear, put in enough dry cotton to fill the ear up, in order to keep the air out.

Sometimes the application of pure olive oil to the ear will relieve it. When the pain is due to a cold which has settled in the ear, it will perhaps be necessary to use warm applications; this may be done, in connection with this remedy, by applying the warm preparations to the outside of the ear and the side of the head or face.

REMEDY

FOR THE RELIEF AND CURE OF CHOLERA MORBUS, DIARRHOEA, CRAMPS, SUMMER COMPLAINT, AND OTHER AILMENTS PECULIAR TO HOT WEATHER.

This remedy will greatly relieve, and in most cases cure the various complaints incident to hot weather. I have put up this combination for a number of years and always found that it gave relief, in a majority of cases, at once. If you are liable to any of the above complaints, have this remedy put up at once and keep it on hand for immediate use in case of sudden attacks. After the first trial, you will be sure to keep it always in the house.

Take

Tincture Rhubarb.
    "   Jamaica Ginger.
    "   Cayenne Pepper
    "   Cinnamon.
Essence Peppermint.
Spirits Camphor.
Paregoric.
Laudanum.

} each ½ ounce.

Mix all together.

Directions for using.

The ordinary dose for adults is from 20 drops to a teaspoonful, according to the severity of the attack. It may be taken upon sugar or in a little sweetened water, either warm or cold; the warm is the best.

The dose may, when necessary, be repeated at short intervals, *but for a few doses only.* Ordinarily take a dose every one to three hours until relieved.

When this remedy is given to children *it must* be used with caution; as it is quite strong and should be used accordingly. There is no better medicine for the purpose when taken properly.

The dose must always be in proportion to age—from two drops upwards. For children, the best way is to add enough sugar to water to make a heavy syrup; then add the required amount of medicine to the syrup. Children will generally take this very nicely. *Make the dose always proportionate to the age.*

PART XVI.

CORNS AND BUNIONS.

What a book might be written on this subject!
There are perhaps few things which cause more excruciating torture, or that come nearer than corns and
bunions, to driving thousands of people crazy.

This condition of things has naturally produced a
very large number of corn and bunion remedies which
have been more or less prominently before the public.
Some of these are no doubt excellent remedies, and if
not *specifics*, will ordinarily perform the work satisfactorily. The manufacturers usually put these preparations up in small parcels, for which they charge an
enormous price, and they have been, as a rule, very
fortunate in drawing money from the people. A
person will not generally stop on price for anything
which affords relief, when suffering from a corn or
bunion.

If the unfortunate victims of corns will try the preparations made after the following recipes and treat the
corns according to instructions, they will positively
secure relief, as I know by many successful trials.

The soreness will be removed from the corns and
bunions, and the corn will come out just as quickly by
the use of this remedy as it can be made to do by any
external application whatever. Do not suffer with
corns any longer, but try the following remedy.

CORN AND BUNION REMEDY

IN

LIQUID FORM.

Take

Flexible Collodion, 6 drachms.
Salicylic Acid, 1½ drachm.
Fluid Extract *India* Hemp, 2 drachms.

Dissolve the salicylic acid in the collodion; then add the fluid extract of India hemp. Shake together and keep *tightly corked*, as it is very volatile. Keep it in a cool place. Never handle it around or near a fire or light, but always at a safe distance from it.

If it should evaporate, as it sometimes does, it can be made all right by adding enough strong sulphuric ether to dissolve the residuum left in the bottle. Stir up the bottom in order to start the solution.

Directions for using.

Do not use this preparation near fire, as it is very inflammable.

Apply the remedy to the corn or bunion with the cork, or a small camel's hair pencil or brush; put on enough to form a coating upon the corn; this can best be accomplished by applying it thin. Allow to dry, then apply a little more, and so on until a thin coating forms on the corn. Do not disturb it, but allow it to get thoroughly dry. The best time to use it is at night, just before retiring.

Repeat this operation two to four times at night. The night after you leave off using it the corn should be thoroughly soaked in *hot* water from 5 to 10 minutes; then wipe off the water and run the thumb nail or point of pen-knife around the outer edge of the corn and gradually raise it up from the outside towards the center until it lifts off.

After you have gone all through the above course and the corn fails to come out, wait a few days, and repeat the same treatment. The number of nights that it should be applied must be determined by the conditions; two to four nights are all that is usually necessary for successful cure. Though the first course of treatment will sometimes prove ineffectual, this should not discourage you ; just wait a few days and try again. Persevere until your success is complete.

I think this remedy when properly used will cure over ninety per cent of cases, and alleviate intolerable agony from corns.

For bunions, just apply the remedy to them every one, two, to three days for a period of from one to three weeks, to take out the soreness. Do not put it on too often or too much at one time.

CORN REMEDY IN FORM OF SALVE.

Inasmuch as some people prefer a corn remedy in this form, I will give them a recipe to make it. They will find this an excellent one; it is in every way just as efficacious as any in the market. In many instances this salve has proved itself to be a specific in relieving, and curing hard and soft corns. It will also give relief to those suffering from a bunion.

Do not hesitate to use this when you are in want of a remedy of this kind, in preference to high priced

preparations of similar character. Make it yourself or
have your druggist put it up from your own recipe.
Take

> Benzoated lard, 6 drachms.
> Salicylic Acid, 2 drachms.
> Pulv. Extract India Hemp, ½ drachm.
> " " Opium, 10 grains.
> Oil Peppermint, 3 drops.
> " Sassafras, 3 drops.
> Glycerine, ½ drachm.
> Simple Ointment, 1 drachm.

Prepare by rubbing the salicylic acid up with the
benzoated lard; then add the oils; rub the extracts up
with the glycerine, and add the simple ointment. Then
rub the two mixtures together until it is a smooth
salve; put in glass or porcelain jar; (do not put in tin
or wood). Keep in cool place, well covered.

Directions for using.

For bunions apply the salve very lightly every night,
or if preferred it may be applied in the morning. Rub
on gently and allow it to remain without being
disturbed ; or it can be put on to a soft piece of cloth
(linen is the best) and laid on to the bunion. Do not
put on too much at one time; the cloth may be held on
by a light bandage. This can be done better at night
than any other time. Follow up until the soreness is
taken out.

For corns apply it at night, with a piece of cloth tied
around the corn ; keep it on through the day. The
ointment must be in contact with the corn. It generally requires from two to four applications, although
sometimes less will do. Soak the corn in hot water for
a few minutes ; then wipe off and run point of pen-knife

or the sharp thumb nail around the outer edge of the corn, and gradually raisé it towards the centre until it comes out.

If the first course proves a failure, try it again.

Soft corns must be treated with the salve, by applying it to the corn lightly. If the corn is very sore, keep cotton over the sore to prevent irritation. Put the salve on the piece of cotton and bind with a light strip of cloth. Have it mild for the first few applications ; continue this for a few days, then intermit for a week ; and so on several times, after which the corn should be well soaked in warm water and taken out as above directed for hard corns. Follow these directions strictly and a cure is certain.

If the corn should become inflamed or irritated in any way by this treatment, stop it, and apply a little of one of the healing ointments on a small piece of cotton. After the inflammation has subsided try the corn salve again. But the salve will generally cure the most tender and obstinate soft corns. When you have a corn which is extremely sore do not handle it much, and do not put on much of any remedy ; as harsh handling will increase the soreness.

When the above preparations, both the liquid and salve, are carefully applied, they seldom fail to relieve the trouble, and generally effect a complete cure. Used occasionally, they will *prevent* corns and bunions.

COMPOUND CAJEPUT.
TOOTHACHE CURE.

There are comparatively few people who have not suffered more or less from toothache. Multitudes therefore, will be able to appreciate a remedy that gives speedy relief. The following remedy will do this every time, when it is possible to stop the toothache without pulling the tooth out.

This formula is one I have used a long time. It has been the means of making a great many people happy by relieving them of the toothache.

If some of my readers should have the toothache they will have my sympathy ; and a recipe to make a preparation which will afford them relief as quick as anything in the world.

Take

Chloroform, ½ ounce.
Oil Cajeput, 3 drachms.
   " Cassia, 1½ drachm.
   " Cloves, 1 drachm.
Camphor Gum, 1 drachm,
Tincture Aconite Root, 1 drachm.
Laudanum, 6 drachms.
Alcohol to make three ounces.

Put camphor gum into a three ounce bottle ; put the oils and other ingredients on the gum ; after all have been added fill the bottle with alcohol and shake up well.

This makes quite a quantity of toothache medicine ; it does not cost much. Keep it tightly corked and it will last a long time ; so that in case of sudden toothache it can be had conveniently. A smaller quantity may be put up ; but keep the proportions the same.

This makes a powerful remedy ; handle it accordingly.

Directions for using.

If the teeth that ache have cavities in them, take a

small piece of cotton and saturate it thoroughly with the remedy ; then insert it into the cavities ; at the same time apply some of the remedy to the gums surrounding the aching teeth.

This may be repeated at short intervals and the cotton replaced by a new and freshly saturated piece. Apply it to the gums ; use the finger.

The bottle in which this remedy is to be kept should be plainly labeled *poison ;* all toothache cures are poisonous, although they are not generally labeled so, because they are put up and sold in such small quantities.

MAGIC NEURALGIA REMEDY.

The following is an excellent preparation for the immediate relief of neuralgia, toothache and rheumatic pains. It is not excelled by any external remedy sold.

I have prepared it for customers hundreds of times, and it always gave immediate relief. It is really a very powerful combination, and yet in no way injurious to use.

The magic of its power seems to be in controlling pain. I never saw anything like it as an external application.

Take

    Camphor Gum, 2 drachms.
    Tincture Cayenne Pepper, 3 drachms.
    Oil Sassafras, 2 drachms.
     " Wormwood, 1 drachm.
     " Origanum, 2 drachms.
    Menthol Chrystals, 20 grains.

Essential Oil Mustard, ½ drachm.
Chloroform, 3 drachms.
Water, 2 drachms.
Alcohol, 4 ounces.

Add the camphor, menthol, chloroform and oils to the alcohol; after they have all been dissolved by shaking them together thoroughly, add the pure water. Keep this medicine tightly corked.

Directions for Using.

In applying this medicine, it should not be forgotten that a little of it will go quite a ways; it should therefore be used lightly over the seat of pain and rubbed on thoroughly. For headache or neuralgia in the head, apply with the fingers to the back part of the head, at the base of the brain, and directly back of the ears; also on the upper forehead and crown of the head. The operation may be repeated at short intervals until relief is obtained.

This remedy will often cure the very worst type of neuralgia; it must be used with some caution, as it is very powerful, although perfectly harmless when used properly.

CHILBLAINS.

This difficulty afflicts a great many people, especially in cold weather. It is naturally aggravated by the changes which take place during winter.

This preparation will relieve and often cure the worst chilblains. I have used the different ones for the complaint in its various stages on different people, for this class of remedies is like any other; one will not serve for all, or in all stages of the difficulty. It might work very satisfactorily with some, but would completely fail with others.

Among these recipes there will no doubt be one that will afford relief and effect a cure in the various cases.

CHILBLAIN REMEDY, NO. 1.

Take
    Tincture Arnica, 1 ounce.
       "   Calandula, 1 ounce.
    Peppermint Water, 1 ounce.
    Alcohol, 1 ounce.
    Pulv. Alum, 2 drachms.

Dissolve the alum in the peppermint water; then add the alcohol and other ingredients.

Directions.

Bathe the affected parts with the above night and morning.

It may be put on very freely until relief is obtained, which will generally be after a few applications. It must be continued long enough to effect a cure, if this be possible with this remedy; when it fails try one of the following: When the chilblains are painful, and there is great soreness and tenderness, the best way to bathe the parts affected is to saturate a small sponge with the remedy and apply it.

CHILBLAIN REMEDY, NO. 2.

This remedy should not be used if the skin is broken, as it would be too strong, and would consequently irritate the sore. After the skin has been healed and the break closed up by a weaker preparation like the preceding, do not delay the use of No. 2, which no doubt will speedily cure the difficulty.

Take

Granulated Muriate Ammonia, ½ ounce.

Pure Water, 4 ounces.

" Muriatic Acid, 2 drachms.

Alcohol, 1½ ounce.

Dissolve the muriate of ammonia in the water; add the muriatic acid to the alcohol; then mix the two solutions together.

Directions for using.

Apply this remedy lightly to the parts affected, night or morning; allow it to dry each time. It may be applied with a soft sponge or old soft cloth. Continue the treatment until the desired effect is produced.

CHILBLAIN REMEDY, NO. 3.

This remedy is especially adapted to chilblains that are badly swollen, and are otherwise in a severe stage.

Take

Tincture Iodine, ½ ounce.

Solution Chlorinated soda, 1½ ounce.

Mix the two together.

Directions for using.

Paint the chilblains night and morning with the solution. Apply it lightly with a camel's hair pencil. It may not be necessary to use it oftener than every other day; follow this up until a cure is effected.

CHILBLAIN REMEDY, NO. 4.

The following recipe makes one of the very best

preparations for chilblains. It seems to afford relief when other remedies have failed to do so. I have seen it perform good work in some very severe cases in which a great many different remedies had been tried without avail.

Take

    Soap Liniment, 2 ounces.
    Oil Cajeput, ½ ounce.
    Tinct. Cantharides, ½ ounce.
    "   Iodine, 2 drachms.
    Alcohol, 1 ounce.

Mix all together.

Apply night and morning, or oftener, if necessary, to control the pain and suffering. It can be used gently, as a liniment.

PART XVII.

REMEDY FOR COLD IN THE HEAD.

NUMBER I.

To relieve and cure a cold that has settled in the head is sometimes very perplexing. It often baffles the skilled physician. Then a person will continue to suffer and submit to the inevitable. This at times produces a terrible condition of the head, until it does seem as though nothing would afford relief.

The following prescription used as a snuff frequently gives immediate relief. I have suggested it a good many times and found that it gave universal satisfaction.

If my readers should require anything of this nature, have the following recipe put up. It may be just the thing for you; it has done good in a thousand cases.
Take

    Finely Pulverized Camphor gum, 2½ drachms.
       "   "   White Sugar, 4 drachms.
    Pulv. Borax, ½ drachm.
    "   Gum Arabic, 2 drachms.
    Oil Wintergreen, 2 drops.
    " Anise Seed, 2 drops.

Rub the powders all together; then add the oils, and rub until the whole is thoroughly mixed.

Directions.

Snuff the powder up the nostrils; use only a small quantity of it in this way once in two to four hours as may be required to relieve the congestion.

The powder should be kept in a tight box, or in a wide mouth bottle tightly corked.

If the congestion is very severe, the snuff may be used for a few times once in every 15 to 20 minutes; then follow at longer periods.

The above recipe makes a small quantity; a larger amount can be made by increasing the amount of the ingredients. A little of this powder goes a good ways, and it is better if not very old.

REMEDY FOR CURING COLD IN THE HEAD.

NUMBER II.

The following formula will also be found very efficacious in relieving and curing cold, catarrh or influenza in the head. In fact, it has very few superiors for this purpose. It is pleasant and agreeable to use.

This is far from being the case with a great many of these remedies. It nearly always affords relief after the first application. Try it and see.

Take

 Finely Pulverized White Sugar, 1 ounce.
   "   "   Camphor gum, ½ ounce.
   "   "   Cubeb Berries, 1½ drachm.
   "   "   Chlorate Potassa, ¼ drachm.
   "   "   Borax, 1 drachm.
 Oil Peppermint, 5 drops.
 " Sassafras, 5 drops.
 " Thyme, 3 drops.

Prepare by mixing the powders all together; then add the oils and rub the whole together until it becomes thoroughly commingled.

Keep in a bottle well corked up, or in a box tightly covered.

Directions for using.

Snuff a small quantity of the powder well up the nostrils, getting it up into the passages, several times a day; the number of times will depend upon the conditions, and will have to be left to the judgment of the user. In acute attacks it will be necessary to use it oftener than chronic cases of long standing. It is comparatively easy to learn how to use the two preceding preparations. It will save time and labor to allow the druggist to put them up for you, as only a small quantity is required.

THROAT AND LUNG REMEDIES.

Probably there is no class of remedies in which more

people are interested than those which will relieve and
cure the different diseases of the throat and lungs,
so prevalent among people living in particular sections
of our country.

The number that are annually claimed as victims of
these diseases almost staggers the mind. It becomes
our duty to do all in our power to stop this terrible
onslaught of the destroyer, and to strengthen the throat
and lungs for the vicissitudes of our climate.

What can we do? I can answer this question with
knowledge obtained from the vast amount of such
cases that I came in contact with in the course of my
professional career.

Invariably I found that the victims of lung troubles
were being slowly but surely carried away, because
they failed to heed nature's first warning.

It is our duty to heed nature's warning, and at once
procure a remedy that relieves the cold or cough which
has settled, and not allow it to go on—as is so often
the case—until some severe throat or lung difficulty is
developed.

If the acute attack is not checked and the natural
forces helped to throw off the disease, there follows one
or more of the various throat and lung difficulties, such
as bronchitis, asthma, hoarseness, croup, tightness in
the chest, difficult breathing, sore throat, pain in the
chest, or some other ailments which can be traced
directly to the neglected cold. How often does it continue until consumption claims another victim?

Much suffering may be avoided if the first symptoms
of a cold are treated with one of the preparations which
can be made after the following recipes.

I know from practical experience that these simple combinations, when taken in time, will do equally as much to relieve the various throat and lung difficulties as any of the so-called wonderful discoveries for which exclusive results are claimed, that prove in the end to be only a myth.

Of course we continue to have new discoveries which are based upon actual scientific principles. These must, however, not be classed with the discoveries on paper that rarely have any semblance of science, but are as worthless as the generality of quack nostrums.

The following preparations I have seen used in a great many cases with the most gratifying results. During my long experience in the handling of medicines, I have put up a great many hundred bottles, and noticed their favorable effects in throat and lung complaints.

COUGH SYRUP.

The following remedy is especially applicable where there exists considerable irritation in the throat, accompanied by a dry hard cough and difficult breathing.

Take

    Syrup Senega, ½ ounce.

      "   Dover Powder, 1 ounce.

      "   Squills, 2 drachms.

      "   Tolu, 1½ ounce.

    Paragoric, ½ ounce.

    Pure Glycerine, 2¼ ounces.

Mix all together. This will make six ounces of the syrup.

Directions for using.

The dose of this syrup for adults is from one to two

teaspoonsful, according to conditions. Take every one to three hours.

If the ailment is very severe, take two teaspoonsful every two hours, for a spell; then take one teaspoonful as often. If the difficulty has somewhat abated, make the intervals longer. Take the last dose just before retiring; this often prevents coughing in the night.

It should be distinctly understood that the age (especially of children) and general health of the person taking the medicine must govern the dose. The severity of the complaint should regulate the intervals in which the medicine may be taken. If this course is systematically adhered to, the disease will succumb to the treatment.

RYE AND ROCK CANDY COMBINATION,

FOR THE RELIEF AND CURE OF COLDS AND COUGHS.

This recipe makes an excellent combination to use in throat and lung difficulties.

It will often break up a cold quicker than anything else that can be used. For a new or recent cold, take it hot before going to bed. It may be used by anybody, old or young, and is pleasant to take.

Take

Pure Rock Candy, 8 ounces.
Water, ½ pint.

Dissolve the rock Candy in the water, by heating it

slightly; when dissolved, strain it: then let it get cold, and add the following:

> Pure Glycerine, 3 ounces.
> Tincture Tolu, 2 drachms.
> Pure Rye Whiskey, ½ pint.

Shake all together; keep well corked.

Directions for using.

A dose is from a teaspoonful to a tablespoonful, or more, according to the severity of the case, and as often as required to relieve, and finally cure, the difficulty.

When desired, Jamaica rum may be used in place of the rye whiskey; this is a matter of taste.

JAMAICA RUM, HONEY AND TAR REMEDY

FOR THE RELIEF AND CURE OF THE VARIOUS

THROAT AND LUNG DISEASES.

This preparation is one of the old reliable ones, which every druggist and a great many outsiders are familiar with.

The formulas differ some; the proportions of the ingredients vary. The following is one that I found to give general satisfaction. It is very soothing and healing.

Take

> Jamaica Rum, ½ pint.
> Pure Strained Honey, ½ pint.
> " Oil Tar, 1 drachm

Mix all together; shake well each time you use it. Dose, from a dessert to a tablespoonful, or more if

necessary to control the difficulty. When administered
to children the dose should be smaller.

COUGH SYRUP FOR CHILDREN.

The following recipé makes a cough syrup for children. It is very simple, yet it is a decidedly efficacious
remedy for colds or coughs, with difficult expectoration,
and the other numerous ailments incidental to taking
cold.

I have put it up a great many times, and positively
know that it makes a remedy which will speedily relieve
and cure a cold, if it is only taken in time, and will
generally prevent a long siege of coughing.

This preparation may be given to children without
any hesitation, as it is very mild, and agreeable to take.
Keep the syrup in cool place.

Take

    Paragoric, ½ ounce.
    Syrup Tolu, ½ ounce.
      " Ipecac, ½ ounce.
      " Senega, 2 drachms.
    Hive Syrup, 2 drachms.

Mix together; keep in bottle well corked.

Directions.

This syrup may be given to children in doses of from
two drops to one teaspoonful, according to age and
symptoms, once in one, two, three, or four hours. For
adults larger doses, of from one teaspoonful to two teaspoonfuls, are necessary.

There can be no set rule for giving this syrup to

children; this must be governed by circumstances. Give at such intervals as may be considered proper for controlling the difficulty.

THROAT AND LUNG BALM.

The following recipe will make a very effective remedy in those acute attacks of cold which cause such irritation in the throat, often accompanied with severe spasmodic coughing.

Take

Syrup Wild Cherry, 1 ounce.
    "   Tolu, 1½   "
    "   Ipecac, ½   "
Fluid Extract Henbane, 1 drachm.
Mucilage Gum Arabic, 1 ounce.
Chloroform, 10 drops.

Mix all together; keep well corked.

Directions for using.

Always shake the medicine together thoroughly before using it.

Dose for an adult, from half to one teaspoonful at intervals of one to three hours, as may be necessary to stop the coughing.

MIXTURE FOR COLDS, COUGHS,

AND ALL

THROAT AND LUNG DISEASES.

The following remedy is another old, reliable, and well tried preparation for throat and lung difficulties.

I have known it to produce extraordinary results in cases of long standing, where other expedients failed. If the reader has a long standing cough this remedy will cure it if not beyond human aid.

Take

Tinct. Benzoin Composition, 2 drachms.
" Blood Root, 2 drachms.
Fluid Extract Ipecac, ½ drachm.
" " Grindilia Robusta, 2 drachms.
Iodide Potassa, 2 drachms.
Water, 4 drachms.
Mucilage Gum Arabic, 1 ounce.
Plain Syrup, 5 ounces.

Prepare by dissolving the Iodide Potassa in the water; add the solution to the plain syrup; then add the mucilage, extracts and tinctures; shake all together.

Directions.

Always shake well before using.

Dose for adults, one teaspoonful every one to four hours according to the symptoms and conditions.

COMPOUND HONEY BALSAM.

The following recipe will make one of the old-fashioned preparations for healing the throat and lungs and curing all diseases of these organs.

This is positively a good remedy. Some people may perhaps think this strange when they notice the composition, and may wonder why they suffer with these diseases when there are so many very good preventives.

But first, try the preparations, now that you need be no longer ignorant of their existence. There are, however, many different constitutions, and all should have remedies to suit their individual systems. For this reason it is necessary to have a variety of remedies. I therefore place some of the most thoroughly tried recipes in this book, to give all an opportunity of securing relief. I trust they will take advantage of it. To make the COMPOUND HONEY BALSAM,

Take

Pure Strained Honey, 3 ounces.
Balsam Fir, 2 drachms.
Tincture Benzoin Comp., 1 drachm.
Fluid Extract Boneset, 4 drachms.
Syrup Tar, 2 ounces.
New England Rum, 3 ounces.

Mix all together; shake well.

Directions.

Always shake well before using.

Dose for an adult from a teaspoonful to a dessert-spoonful. Take as often as necessary to control the ailment. When given to children reduce the dose, according to their age.

COMPOUND LIQUORICE COUGH MIXTURE.

The following is an excellent remedy for throat and lung difficulties; it will sometimes afford relief and effect a cure when other remedies fail.

Do not despair if you have an obstinate cold, but keep trying until you secure the right remedy.

If other things have failed try this remedy.

Take

Compound Liquorice (Brown) Mixture, 3 ounces.

Granulated Muriate Ammonia, 2 drachms.
Syrup Ipecac, 1 ounce.
Fluid Extract Wild Cherry, ½ ounce.
Pure Glycerine, 2 ounces.
Tincture Peruvian Bark Com., 1½ ounce.

Prepare by dissolving the muriate ammonia in the liquorice mixture; then add the other ingredients.

Directions.

Always shake well before using.

Dose for an adult one to two teaspoonsful once in from one to three hours, according to the severity of the complaint.

General Remarks.

In using these Remedies for the throat and lungs, a person must be governed largely by circumstances. When the difficulty is extremely troublesome, half a dose of the medicine may be taken every half hour for a few hours, then increase at intervals so as to get the best results.

It is, however, well to remember that it is never safe to place too much dependence upon a person's own ability to correctly diagnose the disease, unless there is special training for this work. Therefore, whenever there is any doubt whatever in relation to the nature of the ailment, it is decidedly safest to employ a good physician, especially for children.

There is scarcely any limit to the number or character of prescriptions that could be placed here for the relief and cure of throat and lung diseases; but there is no advantage in having too many. Among those I have placed in this work there will be no difficulty in finding one which will relieve and, if possible, cure the ailment.

CATARRH.

How many thousands of people suffer from this malady? what a distressing complaint it is, and how difficult it sometimes is to cure? It is truly remarkable to observe how a great many people allow the disease to go on without making any effort whatever to check it, until it reaches a stage where the organs of the throat and lungs become dangerously diseased; then it is generally too late to effect a cure. At this stage many begin to realize that something is the matter with them, and will then make a great effort to check the onward course of the disease, only to find that they have waited too long. If the matter is taken in hand early in its first stage with some good treatment, and followed up faithfully, it can generally be checked.

Do not allow the system to become exhausted and feeble; when you have a cold in the head, do not allow it to run and take its course, for if you do it will invariably lead to serious catarrhal difficulty. This is the way that the foundation for catarrh is laid.

A great many people suffer from periodical cold in the head, Influenza and Hay fever, causing all the innumerable disagreeable attending conditions, such as acrid watery discharge from the eyes and nose, and painful imflammation of the mucous lining which freequently extends to the throat, with choking and cough-

ing, ringing noises in the head, and fearful headache
—besides numerous other derangements—all of which
might be largely prevented, by resorting to some proper
treatment.

I would suggest to any of my readers who may be
affected as above set forth, to procure at once a remedy
made after one of the following recipes, and see what
good results may be obtained from its use.

COMPOUND MENTHOL SNUFF,

FOR THE RELIEF AND CURE OF COLD IN THE HEAD, INFLUENZA, HAY FEVER AND CATARRH.

Take
    Finely pulverized Cubeb Berries, 1 drachm.
      "   " White Sugar, 2 ounces.
      "   " Menthol Crystal, 12 grains.
    Impalpable Powder Boracic Acid, ¼ drachm.
    Oil Wintergreen, 10 drops.

Prepare by rubbing the powders all together; then
add the oil, and continue rubbing them until all are
thoroughly commingled; keep in bottle corked tightly
or in a box securely covered.

Directions for using.

This powder should be used as a snuff several times
a day, snuffing it up the nostrils. In acute attacks it may
be used often, in small quantities. It should be drawn
up well into the passages as often as may be necessary
to control the difficulty.

The above remedy works like magic. In some cases
of long standing catarrh it has produced remarkable
effects. The result will in some instances surprise you.

When persisted in it will often bring about a complete cure, as I know from personal knowledge.

BEGY'S CATARRH REMEDY.

The following remedy for relieving and curing catarrhal difficulty in its various stages, anybody can use with confidence. I have seen its results for years, and know that by its use some very bad cases of catarrh have been greatly benefited and some cured. It will always give relief, and when used occasionally it will prevent the development of catarrh in people who would otherwise naturally be troubled with it. It has cured where other remedies failed. It is very simple, effective and inexpensive. It is certainly worth a trial.

Take

Pulverized Chlorate Potassa, 5 grains.
" Borax, 10 grains.
Granulated Muriate Ammonia, 8 grains.
Pure Carbolic Acid, 8 grains.
Peppermint Water, 1½ ounce.
Distilled Extract Witch Hazel, 1 ounce.
Pure Glycerine, 1 ounce.
Pure Water, 4½ ounces.

Dissolve the ammonia, borax and chlorate potassa in the water; then add the other ingredients; shake together; keep in cool place tightly corked.

Directions for using.

Procure at the Drug store a small nasal douche ; the one which serves the purpose nicely is made by getting a small nasal piece, made of glass or hard rubber, and a small vial in which the nasal piece should be placed. This you will notice makes a very good little douche, and it has the advantage of not being expensive; You can if you prefer it, buy the small douche all complete. When the vial, as above suggested, is used, it should be partly filled with the remedy; then place the nasal piece inside. Then put the nose piece to the nostril and draw the liquid up into the head. About 2 teaspoonsful of the remedy should be used each time on each side of the head. Draw the remedy up into the head equally through both nostrils. It may be used once or twice a day, according to the conditions and severity of the complaint.

If the remedy smarts very much, as it will perhaps the first few times it is used, or if it irritates the passages, reduce it by adding pure water to it until it causes no unpleasant sensation in the nostrils; first fill the vial partly with the remedy; then fill up with pure water; or the preparation may be reduced before it is applied at all.

When the douche is used, partly fill the tube with the remedy in same way, and apply as above, about 2 teaspoonsful at a time.

The above remedy will positively relieve and perhaps entirely cure this distressing and disagreeable disease. Hardly any ailment is more obnoxious than a bad case of catarrh in the advanced stages.

Sometimes it may be necessary, in connection with this treatment, to take some good constitutional medicine; in fact I have always suggested this in long standing cases of catarrh, especially when the blood is deteriorated, which is generally the case in a chronic disease. It is now quite generally conceded that in a majority of cases catarrh of long duration must be treated both locally and constitutionally.

PART XVIII.

There is perhaps no better remedy to take as a constitutional medicine for catarrh than some sarsaparilla compound. I always found that the compound made from the following recipe would work very satisfactorily when it is found necessary to use constitutional treatment in connection with the local one. Do not fail to try the BLOOD PURIFIER.

BLOOD PURIFIER,

NUMBER 1.

Take
Iodide Potassa, 2 drachms.
Fluid Extract Rhubarb, 2 drachms.
   "   "   Ginger Root, 1 drachm.
   "   "   Senna Leaves, ½ ounce.
Syrup Sarsaparilla Composition, 7 ounces.

Dissolve the iodide potassa in the syrup sarsaparilla; then add the fluid extracts.

Directions.

Shake well each time before taking it.

Dose for an adult, from one to two teaspoonsful three times a day, with a wine glass of water, one hour after each meal.

The quantity to be taken must be regulated by the condition of the complaint.

When given to children the dose should be according to their age.

The above COMPOUND SARSAPARILLA is an excellent blood purifier; it is by all odds a better remedy than the majority of the so-called blood purifiers that are lauded up to the sky.

The above remedy and also the one following, have no superior for rejuvenating the system; they will without a shadow of doubt cure just as many ailments as any of the so-called new and wonderful discoveries.

When the Number One Blood Purifier does not answer the purpose try the following, which may agree with the case better. I have frequently found where one failed the other worked very nicely. Try them and you will get just as good if not better results from these remedies than from others which cost twice the amount of money.

BLOOD PURIFIER,

NUMBER 2.

This blood remedy will build the system up and cure a great many of the various complaints which are brought on by the blood being in an impure state. It is an established fact that there cannot be good health when the blood is in an impure condition.

Take

Iodide Potassa, 2 drachms.
Bromide Potassa, 4 drachms.
Pure Water, 4 ounces.

Simple Syrup, 3 ounces.

Fluid Extract Senna, ½ ounce.

"   "   Sarsaparilla Compound, 1 ounce.

Best Whiskey, 3 ounces.

Prepare by dissolving the iodide and bromide of potassa in the water; then add the simple syrup, fluid extracts and whiskey.

Shake all together; keep tightly corked.

Directions.

Dose for an adult is from one to two teaspoonfuls of this medicine three times a day, with about a wine glass full of water.

It should be taken about one hour after meals.

When this medicine is given to children the dose must be according to their ages.

The number of times that it should be given through the day must be regulated by the wants of the system.

BEEF, IRON AND WINE.

Where is the person who has not heard of it?

There are few names with which the public is more familiar than this preparation, and yet they do not know anything about its composition. I am inclined to think a formula for making it will be highly appreciated, and be of considerable value to some of my readers.

There is probably no one preparation that is used with greater satisfaction for a very large number of complaints, and the demand for it seems to be continually increasing.

When a tonic is required to build up the run-down

system there are thousands of people who resort to this preparation. I have seen some splendid results follow the use of it.

It is very mild and agreeable to take, on which account a great many people can use it without the least unpleasant effects; and extremely good results follow, where the more powerful or stronger iron combinations could not be tolerated.

This preparation is especially indicated in that low state of the system to which many people are subject who have had malaria; also for loss of appetite, languor, and after a long siege of sickness where the recovery of strength and vitality is slow and where it often seems to the patient that they will never get strong again.

In fact it may be used to good advantage at nearly any time that something is required to restore the tone and vigor of the system. How many people suffer from a low state of vitality? They can be numbered by the thousands. They go through this life in a half-starved condition, and their system is continually craving for something. What is it? It is some such preparation as this that is wanted to rejuvenate and build up the system of thousands of people who cannot eat a meal without great distress, and who would give a great deal to be able to eat heartily and feel well; to be able to digest what they eat and not have to submit to the pangs of dyspepsia, a complaint that most people in America suffer from more or less. I have added below a recipe for making a DYSPEPSIA COMPOUND, to which I refer those who suffer from this distressing complaint.

I ask those afflicted to give this preparation of Beef,
Iron and Wine a trial. It may be just what your
system needs. It can do no harm. It can also be used
in conjunction with the Dyspepsia Compound with the
happiest results.

Beef, Iron and Wine can be made after the following formula for very much less cost than is charged for
it by the dealers. The market at the present time is
flooded with preparations called Beef, Iron and Wine.
I am compelled to say that a great many of them are
made up of very poor quality of material; especially
is this so as regards the quality of sherry wine used in
making them. Then again others use a very small
amount of beef, which is often of an inferior quality.

Some pharmacists that make this excellent and valuable medicinal preparation claim to use fresh beef. I
have tried this, but with unsatisfactory results; consequently I gave up using the fresh beef, and ever after
confined myself to the use of a first-class quality of
the Extract of Beef.

In making this preparation it is absolutely essential
to have good quality of material; nothing else should
be used; for if it is prepared from poor or inferior
material the finished product must necessarily be of an
inferior quality. This would lay my recipe open to
strong condemnation; so I wish to impress upon my
readers the importance of using only good materials.
There are perhaps very few things in the line of
medicinal preparations that have deteriorated in
quality as much as this preparation in the last few
years. But by making your own preparation after my
recipe you will see just what it is made of, and know

that you are getting the best quality of Beef, Iron and Wine for the least money.

I desire to be rightly understood in this matter. I do not make the claim that my recipe will make the best possible preparation, for no doubt a great many capable druggists make equally as good. But I do claim that if you have this recipe you will be able to make a first-class Beef, Iron and Wine at a cost no greater than is generally charged for an inferior preparation. Thus you will save many times the price of this volume.

I have used the following formula a number of years in making this preparation and have sold hundreds of bottles of it; and I speak with a full and thorough knowledge of its merits.

The simple elixir called for in the recipe is a solution of aromatics. It gives to the Beef, Wine and Iron a pleasant and agreeable flavor. It can be had at any drug store, as well as the other ingredients.

I have simplified this recipe, so that it will be a very easy matter to prepare the Beef, Iron and Wine.

Take

    Best Quality Extract Beef, 1 ounce.
    Pure Glycerine, 4 ounces.
    Simple Syrup, 4 ounces.
    Aquæ Ammonia, 1 drachm.
    Simple Elixir, 4 ounces.
    Ammoniated Citrate Iron, 6 drachms.
    Hot Water, 2 ounces.
    Fluid Extract Lovage, ½ drachm.
    Good quality Sherry Wine, 1¼ pint.

Prepare as follows :

In buying the ingredients from your druggists have

the glycerine, ammonia, syrup and simple elixir put together. Then have the fluid extract lovage, put with the sherry wine. The lovage can be left out, if desired; it, however, adds very much to the character of the preparation, by giving it that peculiar flavor so generally looked for. Have the citrate of iron put up separately in paper. Put the different ingredients together by dissolving the citrate of iron in the hot water. After it is dissolved, add the solution to the sherry wine. Then dissolve the extract of beef in mixture of simple syrup, elixir and ammonia. This can very readily be done by mixing all together in a bottle that will hold about a quart and shaking frequently for a period of an hour or two.

When it has been dissolved, add the two mixtures together, and you will have the Beef, Iron and Wine then completed. Not a very difficult thing to make, after all, is it?

It must now be left standing for two days. If at the end of this time there should be a precipitate (sediment) at the bottom, pour off the clear liquid from above; or it may be filtered through filtering paper.

This recipe makes about a quart of the preparation.

Directions for using.

Dose: one teaspoonful to a tablespoonful, before or after meals; or it may be taken every 2 or 3 hours, if necessary, according to conditions.

DYSPEPSIA.

What untold despair and suffering this complaint implies, will never be known to those who enjoy vigorous digestive powers. It is generally called the *Great American Complaint.* Indeed it is a fact, that very few people in this country are entirely free from it.

If ever a person is justified in giving way to hopelessness it is when suffering from the ravages and tortures of dyspepsia. But the sufferers from this distressing complaint have generally only themselves to blame; for in the majority of cases it is brought on by abusing nature.

It should not be forgotten that nature is a stern and exacting judge ; if she is slow at times, she is none the less sure to demand a hearing. Therefore all should beware and pay heed to warnings that nature gives from time to time. If these are disregarded, poor health, suffering, despondency, unhappiness and often despair ensue.

I have seen a great deal of this suffering from dyspepsia and indigestion, and will say to those afflicted that they must make up their minds to apply themselves to some remedy which will meet their case, and use it faithfully until they get relieved. This, however, will have to be assisted by a judicious diet. You must not eat food of any kind that will distress you ; it is positively necessary to abstain from such food before you can expect to get any relief. I have learned by experience that it is a grave error of some writers and physicians of prominence to advocate certain rules to govern all cases. This I declare to be positively wrong in theory as well as in practice. The problem can only be solved properly and correctly by each individual having his own rules to go by, and to eat according to what he finds to agree with him. I am aware that this may be open to a certain amount of discussion, on the ground that so few people will voluntarily suffer any deprivation for themselves. Yet after a short experience of dyspepsia, they will be sufficiently impressed with the serious importance of doing so; and will learn to eat only such nutritious food, and in such quantity as will agree with the stomach.

Following will be found a recipe for making the COMPOUND DYSPEPSIA POWDER.

If all dyspeptics will use this remedy, and follow the above suggestions, I venture to say they will be pleased with the result.

This subject is one that cannot be thoroughly discussed in this work. What I have said must suffice.

I have put up the following preparation many times, and know it has cured some very bad cases of dyspepsia and indigestion. I never have been more pleased with the beneficial effects of any of my preparations. It has given such immediate relief in some cases that the gratification derived from this source was very pleasant and refreshing in the ups and downs of every day life.

To prepare the Dyspepsia Compound:

Take

    Pulv. Cinnamon, ½ drachm.
    Pulv. Jam. Ginger, 1½ drachm.
    Pure Sub. Nitrate Bismuth, 2 drachms.
      "   Prepared Chalk,   2   "
      "   Bicarbonate Soda,   2   "
    Pure pulv. Pepsin, 1½ drachm.
      "   "   Gum Arabic, 1½ drachm.

Mix all together, and keep in a wide mouthed bottle, well corked.

Directions.

In having this recipe put up have your druggist weigh out for a sample dose 20 grains. This is equal to about a half teaspoonful in bulk of the powder.

This quantity may be taken as a dose three times a day right after, or with the meals. It can be taken in a small quantity of water, or with sugar and water. Dose for an adult is about ½ teaspoonful of the powder, and the dose for children in proportion to their age. The above preparation is also an excellent remedy for bowel difficulties, such as summer complaints and diarrhœa.

In the use of this and other preparations in severe cases, do not delay for a moment; but go to your druggist and have the recipe put up at once. This will insure proper compounding, and the remedy can be used with confidence.

I have endeavored to make everything so plain throughout this work, that the materials can generally be put up together by any intelligent person.

CONCLUSION.

It is the earnest wish and hope of the author that everybody who reads this book will be better off for having done so, and that its readers may gain knowledge which will be invaluable to them.

" ALL IS WELL THAT ENDS WELL."

INDEX.

256   *Index.*

www.ingramcontent.com/pod-product-compliance
Lightning Source LLC
Chambersburg PA
CBHW020529270326
41927CB00006B/499